Allergy
and
Your Child

By the same author

A PARENT'S GUIDE TO CHILDREN'S ALLERGIES

Allergy and Your Child

Emile Somekh, M.D.

HARPER & ROW, PUBLISHERS
New York · Evanston · San Francisco · London

FIRST EDITION

Designed by Gwendolyn O. England

Library of Congress Cataloging in Publication Data

Somekh, Emile.
   Allergy and your child.
   Bibliography: p.
   1. Pediatric allergy. I. Title.
RJ399.A4S56   618.9′29′7   73–14291
ISBN: 0–06–013969–2

This book is a tribute to Vincent J. Fontana, M.D.
—a teacher and a friend.

Contents

Acknowledgments

The author is indebted to many associations and corporations who have had a part in the development of this book. Appreciation is extended to:

The American Dietetic Association, Beech-Nut Company, Nabisco Company, Cellu Products, and The United Fruit Company for their recipes.

Cooper Laboratories, Inc. for their pamphlet "You and Your Asthma."

A-H Robins for their pamphlets "How to Desensitize a Car for the Allergy Patient," "How to Reduce the Allergic Load for the Allergy-Prone Infant," "How to Desensitize a Room," "What to Do When the Pet Must Go," "Taming the Outdoors for the Allergic Child," and "Building a Model House for the Atopic Child."

The American Academy of Pediatrics for their pamphlet "Breathing Exercises for Asthmatic Children."

Breon Laboratories for their breathing and postural drainage exercises.

The Association of Convalescent Homes and Hospitals for Asthmatic Children for their lists of camps and rehabilitation centers.

Drs. Jerome Glaser, Irwin Rappaport, Gourdji Raby, Fouad Mouallem, and Harvey Wolf for suggestions, assistance, and advice.

Miss Josephine Dimino for her extremely helpful collaboration.

My wife and children for their enthusiasm and cooperation in preparing this book.

Preface

With so many books written for parents and general practitioners about the different allergies of their children and patients, why write a new one? I have three good reasons for doing so.

1. Bringing up children is a difficult job; bringing up allergic children is more difficult because of free advice given by grandmothers, well-intentioned neighbors, and insufficiently trained physicians. To avoid misinformation, some basic facts about how allergy develops and how to cope with it through diet and environmental control should come in handy to the parents as well as to the general practitioner who is helping them in raising "atopic" children, that is, children prone through heredity to develop allergies.

2. Allergy in a child is not purely a sensitivity to an allergen; it is rather a time- and place-linked series of phenomena influenced by emotion. The heredity of the child, his age, his environment, as well as the kind of upbringing he gets, determine to a large extent the type and intensity of his allergy. As a consequence, any allergic disease in a child does not manifest itself as a set of known symptoms because the internal organs of the child communicate with each other in a language which the child finds hard to understand, and therefore difficult to express. The result of this lack of communication and difficulty in expression is a number of misconceptions about the causes of allergy and the influence of emotions on it.

3. Allergy has now become the leading chronic disease of babies and children and needs quick, efficient treatment. If it is left un-

treated, it may lead to asthma, emphysema, and untimely death. The right time to treat it is when it starts—during early life.

On occasion, I have found it necessary to mention the names of drugs, clothing, furniture, summer resorts, or vacation areas. This is not intended to promote their sale or use, but merely to simplify the management of a complex problem.

At intervals, the book may contain repetitions and pure pediatrics. This is intentional; it is done to make the task of a busy parent less onerous.

Emile Somekh, M.D.

Science can never be a closed book. It is like a tree, ever growing, ever reaching new heights. Occasionally the lower branches, no longer giving nourishment to the tree, slough off. We should not be ashamed to change our methods; rather we should be ashamed never to do so.

Charles V. Chapin

1 An Introduction to Baby Allergy

1. One out of every seven people in the United States suffers from an allergic disease.

2. Children with allergies lose 36 million days from school every year and spend about 13 million days in bed because of their allergies.

3. Children with allergies require an average of three times as many medical visits as do those suffering from other types of illnesses.

4. Allergy has now become the leading chronic disease of children.

Fact Sheet, Allergy Foundation of America

ATOPY, OR PREDISPOSITION TO ALLERGY

An atopic baby or a baby born to allergic parents is different from other babies in that he inherits certain characteristics, one of which is a tendency to manufacture an excess of a certain antibody called *reagin* or *IgE*. This antibody may bring about in the atopic child an allergic disease, such as hay fever or asthma, should he be exposed to allergens. Allergens are substances—such as milk, dust, or pollen —found in the natural environment of the atopic child, while antibodies are substances formed in the body of the child to protect him against the harmful effects of these allergens.

But IgE is different from all other antibodies in that it does not protect the atopic child against allergens. In fact, it creates trouble for him by fighting them. In the fight, a chemical by the name of *histamine* is released in certain organs of the body. If it is released in the skin the child gets hives or eczema; if it is released in the nose, he gets hay fever or allergic rhinitis; and if it is released in the chest he gets asthma.

But how does one determine whether a child is allergy prone (atopic) or not? Clinically, it is easy to recognize the manifestations of the main allergic diseases, but it is more difficult to determine their cause. This requires a careful history, an examination by a doctor, and skin testing. A recent discovery called Rast (radio allergosorbent test) may enable physicians to determine in vitro if a child's serum contains antibodies against specific allergens of clinical importance to eliminate the variables inherent in skin testing.

ATOPY AND HEREDITY

Even though hay fever and asthma may be found among dogs and horses, atopy is considered in human genetics as one of the inheritable traits of the human race. Therefore, a person who is allergic and decides to get married should consider these two questions: (1) Should I get married at all and let an innocent partner share my burden? (2) If I do get married, should I have children and possibly see them develop allergies?

Such a person must realize that although he has a trait that is transmitted with mathematical regularity from generation to generation by means of a "gene" or a unit of inheritance, this "gene" is wrapped in a package that will act in one of two ways. It may "open up" and cause disease when exposed to allergens, or it may remain harmlessly "closed" if it is not exposed to allergens. This fact alone should be reassuring to the future parent, because his children can be made to avoid disease by avoiding allergens. Furthermore, if the allergic parent is a woman, pregnancy will not change her status or interfere with her desensitization program.

If the allergic parent is a man, he must not have mixed feelings on the subject. He should keep in mind that his wife chose him for the sum total of all his qualities, and that his good qualities probably outweigh a hereditary tendency over which he has no control whatsoever. Lastly, when the child is born, the loving care that both parents give him is far more important to a healthy upbringing than his atopic heredity.

As a case in point, John Smith is thirty-two years old and has suffered from hay fever all his life. He is married to Anne Jones, twenty-six, who has suffered from eczema all her life. They have five children: John Jr., eight, has no allergies whatsoever; Beatrice, six years old, suffers from seasonal hay fever; Joan, five years old, suffers from eczema and food allergies; Maureen, three, suffers from bronchial asthma; and George, two years old, suffers from a chronic cough.

This particular family was chosen to illustrate heredity in allergy. It shows that if the father and mother have allergies, their children are apt to develop allergies; that these children do not inherit specific allergies but only a predisposition to develop any one of the allergic ailments; that not all children born to two allergic parents develop allergies, but only about 70 percent of them; that allergy in children sometimes does not develop as a clear-cut allergic disease, but may manifest itself as a vague symptom (as in the case of George's cough). If John (who does not have allergies) marries a girl who is also free of allergies, their children will still have a chance of developing an allergy, because John carries hidden in him the allergy gene. Because of thousands of years of intermarriage, most people carry the allergy gene to some extent. If exposed long enough to powerful allergens, practically anyone will develop some allergic manifestations.

THE ALLERGIC PATTERN

An atopic baby or child usually develops allergic symptoms in a predictable fashion. During his first year, his problems relate to foods, skin rashes, and basic immunizations. His second year may be full of upper respiratory infections brought about by exposure to the outside world. In his third year, his home environment starts to catch up with him and give him trouble; his bedroom becomes his main source of allergies. His fourth year is neither/nor; that is, he is not old enough to go to school and he is not young enough to be kept inside. That is why his life belongs to the nursery (where his problems would be similar to those he will encounter later in school), or back yard with its potential allergens. His fifth and sixth years create problems that pertain to traveling to school, attending school, having summer vacations, and going to camp.

But suppose the atopic child does not follow the pattern we have traced for him and starts wheezing in the early days of his life? What can we do then? We have to accept the fact that there is always a possibility that an allergic disorder may start at any age. That is why Chapters 7 and 8, on bronchial asthma, are not age-related.

KEEPING THE ATOPIC BABY WELL

An atopic child does not necessarily develop allergies, because allergy can sometimes be prevented. The following hints to prevent baby and child allergy should be applied while the atopic baby is still in the womb, during the time of his delivery, during his early days, and later on in life.

While in the Womb

Some drugs and foods should be avoided by the allergic mother during her pregnancy. A few drugs are contraindicated in all pregnant women because of their adverse effect on the unborn baby. These are the cytotoxic drugs, the central nervous system depressants, tetracyclines, the anticoagulants, and so forth. The allergic mother who may be using penicillin and antihistamines should take these two drugs only when needed, and with a prescription. Desensitizing injections, however, may be given to such a mother during her pregnancy, provided special care is taken to avoid reactions.

The foods that an allergic mother should avoid during pregnancy are the highly sensitizing ones, such as shellfish, chocolate, and nuts. None of these foods is essential to the nutrition of the atopic baby while he is in the womb.

During Delivery

The obstetrician who delivers an atopic baby must be made aware of the potential dangers inherent in certain drugs used for anesthesia during the delivery period, as well as the dangers of certain antibiotics used after delivery to prevent infection. Among the latter, penicillin deserves special attention.

During the Early Days

Even though colds and respiratory infections are rare during the first few weeks, they acquire importance because they may lead to bronchiolitis and croup. To avoid them, all nonessential visitors— such as neighbors, photographers, salesmen of baby furniture, and so forth—should be kept away from the mother while she is in the hospital, or later in the home, and under no circumstances should they be allowed to touch or fondle the baby. This means that such a baby needs constant supervision by his mother; adequate help for the house chores might be required for weeks or even months, depending on the financial status and physical strength of the mother.

During the Early Months

Proper feeding during the early months is important to prevent food allergies. Allergic babies are born one of a kind, and their food peculiarities have to be recognized and respected. It follows that the problem in feeding such a baby entails more than simply buying and preparing his meals. It means making of his mealtime a healthy and a happy event, unmarred by an allergic reaction that may be expressed by vomiting, gases, or diarrhea. Furthermore, the allergic baby's foods must be made to meet not only his physiological needs but his emotional ones as well. Knowing the kinds of foods that he prefers is important; a baby recognizes instinctively the foods he can safely eat by their odors, flavors, texture, and consistency, and takes pleasure in eating them. He usually avoids the foods that may cause trouble.

Proper feeding of the atopic baby, as well as food alergy, will be dealt with in detail in Chapter 2.

During the First Year

Regular pediatric checkups during the first year should be done to see whether the atopic baby is normal in every respect, that is, that he does not suffer from a heart anomaly, malnutrition, anemia, stunted growth, a hearing or a visual defect. Any one of these diseases could enhance, protract, or complicate his allergies.

Should the atopic infant fall acutely ill, he may need besides the above-mentioned routine office checkups, all or some of the laboratory work-up listed in this chapter.

Later on in Life—The Environment

1. An atopic child must live in a quiet home. He should sleep ten to twelve hours a night and have a nap in the afternoon. His household should be free from emotional strife.

2. The bedroom must be made dust-free. Family pets must never be introduced into it. It must be kept free of bacteria, smoke, polluted air, or odors, through the installation of special electronic devices that purify its air.

3. Control of the outdoor life of the child can be accomplished by keeping him away from bees, insects, poison ivy plants, as well as the ragweed plant. While being outdoors, the child must avoid

becoming overheated or suddenly chilled, because extreme changes in temperatures can lower his resistance to allergies.

Other Miscellaneous Tips

1. Bathing and clothes: Bath oils and afterbath lotions must not be applied too heavily or too frequently on the skin of the baby. A damp cloth should be used to clean the baby's face—no soap. Wool clothing should be avoided during the first year. New clothes should be washed thoroughly to remove any excess dye or other chemicals that have been used in the finishing process.

2. Babysitting: In case the mother of a baby has to be out for an entire day or evening, or an even more extended period of time, the baby-sitter should know:

(a) The telephone number at which the person responsible for the child may be reached; the telephone number of the police, the fire department, the next-door neighbors, the nearest hospital, and the pediatrician of the baby.

(b) A list of the baby's allergies; his likes, his dislikes, his fears; his special characteristics; his favorite TV programs.

(c) The baby's medicine, and how it should be given; specific instructions on what medicines *not* to give the baby, such as aspirin, penicillin, etc.

A baby-sitter must be a healthy person who does not arrive with a cold, does not smoke or take drugs. She must not delegate a friend to take her place, or fall asleep while on the job. Above all, she must have a stable family background, with experience in raising children, and be endowed with lots of heart and common sense.

Emotional Maturity

Of all the instructions on how to keep an allergic child well, the most important one concerns itself with his emotional maturity. A child living with air-purifying gadgets, ready-made allergy-free clothing and furniture, allergy-free camps and vacation areas, and so forth, will probably have an easy and healthy life. However, the parents of such a child must guard against giving him a purely materialistic upbringing. An atopic child who can only thrive by using artificial controls and mechanical devices may idolize the artifacts and gadgets that help him survive. That is why he must be provided with spiritual motivation, religious faith, service of humanity, and active involvement in the affairs of the community must form an integral part of his upbringing to prevent a possible aggravation of his allergies through emotional conflict.

A child who is in need of all the above-mentioned precautions may be hard to accept and love—but acceptance and love are the elements that will instill confidence in him and guide him to health and emotional maturity.

Laboratory Work-up

These are the necessary laboratory examinations that a child may need: a urine examination, serology in mother and child, CBC (complete blood count) for the form of RBC (Red Blood Cells) and its hemoglobin content, and a tine test every two years.

The tine test is one of several important tests used by the general practitioner to detect tuberculosis. Its purpose is not to give immunity against tuberculosis, just to detect it. It is done with a small plastic instrument, one end of which contains four small points or tines coated with testing material. These points are pressed against the forearm for a second or two. Two to three days later, the forearm has to be examined by the doctor for the results of the test. A positive reaction is not unusual, and does not mean that the child has tuberculosis. It means that he has tuberculosis antibodies in his body. The chances are that these antibodies are caused by dead germs which will cause no damage, but a chest X ray is needed to clear the diagnosis. If the reaction is negative, the child has no tuberculosis antibodies in his body now, and the test should be repeated every two years. Tuberculosis is important to detect because it is not only curable, but because it may be accompanied by a chronic cough like that caused by an allergy.

No skin-testing for allergies is usually necessary during the first year of life, even though the child may be suffering from allergies, because food allergies are diagnosed clinically, and inhalant allergies usually develop after two years of age.

2 The Problems of the Atopic Baby During His First Year

FEEDING

A Historical Introduction

The ancient Egyptians, the Babylonians, and the Greeks described hives and stomach upsets caused by eating eggs or fish. Hippocrates diagnosed milk allergy, and prescribed special diets for it. Eight hundred years ago, Moses Maimonides gave detailed food recipes for asthmatic children. More recently, Willis and Salter described asthma caused by drinking wine, milk, malt liquor, or eating cheese and nuts. The list of doctors who have suspected food as a cause of allergy through improper feeding whether in the early months of life or later on is very long, and extends into the present day.

Improper feeding is a term used to denote wrong feeding techniques or the use of foods which are inappropriate to the age of a baby or to his health requirements. This sort of feeding may cause or precipitate allergies to certain foods in case these foods are highly allergenic. Early feeding of these foods promotes their absorption in an incompletely digested form through an intestine which may not have matured.

The foods which should be withheld for a few months because

they are potentially dangerous are nuts, chocolate, eggs, fish, shellfish, corn, tomatoes, fresh juices, and strawberries.

The first food that should be given to a baby is milk. It is a nutritious and healthy food. Its proteins are high in biological value and are far superior to those derived from soybeans, wheat, corn, or rice. The healthiest kind of milk that a baby can have is breast milk.

Breastfeeding the Atopic Baby

An atopic baby has a natural right to the milk of his mother. He should be breastfed, because this makes him less susceptible to infections or allergies. Furthermore, breast milk is clean, needs no refrigeration or warming, is easily available, is cheap, satisfies the sucking impulse of the baby, and provides physical and mental satisfaction to the mother.

A mother who breastfeeds her allergic baby should be adequately fed. Fresh fruits, vegetables, meats, butter, and milk should be given to her in abundance.

Here are a few hints for the breastfeeding mother, in case the atopic baby is a firstborn and the mother has not yet learned the technique.

1. While feeding the baby, the mother may prefer to lie down on her side with the baby resting on her arm. The nipple touches his cheek, and instinct will make him turn his head to search for it.

2. While nursing, the mother must make certain that the baby has the areola—the dark circular area around the nipple—in his mouth, so that his gums squeeze the places that contain milk.

3. Though the baby usually gets most of the milk in five minutes of steady nursing, because he enjoys sucking he may want to nurse for a longer period of time. There is no need, however, to nurse him for longer than twenty to thirty minutes.

4. Until the milk supply is well established, the mother may find that she has to nurse her baby at both breasts at each feeding. If so,

she must alternate the breast she gives him first so that one breast doesn't become overly tender.

Learning the art of relaxed breastfeeding and enjoying it takes time and patience, and the longer the child is breastfed, the better are his chances to be healthy allergy-wise.

Hazards of Breastfeeding the Atopic Baby

Although most doctors agree that breastfeeding is superior to bottlefeeding in preventing allergies, some hazards are inherent in breastfeeding because many drugs are excreted in breast milk. These are:

1. Allergenic antimicrobials, such as penicillin, which may sensitize a breastfed baby even when taken in small quantities by the mother. A mother being treated with penicillin should not breastfeed her baby.

2. Some substances that are excreted in breast milk in exceptionally large amounts. These are the chemicals that contain mercury, bromide, iodine, alcohol, ether, phenobarbital, and oral contraceptives.

3. Some exceptionally potent drugs, which, even though excreted in small quantities in mother's milk, are dangerous nevertheless. These are the steroids, the anticoagulants, and the radioactive chemicals.

4. Drugs that may reach high concentrations in breast milk because the mother cannot eliminate them from her system due to a disease of the kidney.

5. Other drugs that cause harm to the atopic as well as the normal baby because they are neutralized by breast milk. A prime example is Sabin vaccine, which loses some of its potency in a breastfed baby, atopic or otherwise. Breastfeeding should be withheld for some days before the vaccine is given.

Bottlefeeding—the Formula

Breast milk contains all the ideal nutritional substances necessary for the optimal growth of a baby. Nevertheless, a lot of city women who work and have no time for breastfeeding find it convenient to substitute cow's milk. This is inexpensive, easy to procure, and nourishing. Cow's milk, however, is not the ideal food for a baby. It is a food intended for the optimal growth of a calf—a baby animal whose nutritional needs are quite different from those of a human baby.

A baby who is fed cow's milk should be given the closest approximation to breast milk by means of an adequate formula prescribed by a pediatrician. A formula is some combination of ingredients made of cow's milk, water, and sugar. Cow's milk as sold in the market comes in different forms: as raw milk in a bottle, evaporated milk, pasteurized milk, ready-to-use milk-based formula, homogenized milk, half-skimmed milk, skimmed milk and powdered milk. The pediatrician will choose the kind of milk most suited to the needs of the baby and will prescribe it. The sugar to be used is the ordinary granulated white sugar, because it is easily digested and not allergenic. Corn syrup is to be avoided because it is highly allergenic.

A formula may be well tolerated by the baby, or it may present problems caused by enzyme deficiencies or allergy to milk.

Milk Intolerance Due to Enzyme Deficiency

Some children cannot tolerate milk because they do not possess the special enzyme necessary to digest lactose, which is the sugar present in milk. Such children develop colic, vomiting, diarrhea, and constipation.

Milk Intolerance Caused by Allergy

The incidence of allergy to cow's milk varies among atopic babies from 1 to 6 percent, depending on the point of view of the author who is compiling the statistics. Such a high incidence is accounted for by the relatively huge amount of cow's milk a baby is made to consume while his intestines are still immature and unable to digest the relatively elevated amount of casein found in cow's milk as compared to that found in mother's milk.

Milk allergy is often incorrectly diagnosed, and a history alone does not constitute proof of its existence. However, great clinicians like Hippocrates were able to diagnose it, considering the following symptoms as indicative of milk allergy: frequent vomiting, diarrhea, canker sores in the mouth, eczema, hives, rhinitis, and asthma. Today we cannot do much better than they did.

Because vomiting and diarrhea, which are the two cardinal symptoms of this disease, are present in many illnesses of the early months of life, they deserve to be dealt with in detail here.

Vomiting

Early vomiting may occur immediately after a bottle feeding, or half an hour later, and consist of plain milk, curdled milk, milk mixed with mucus, blood, or bile. This type of vomiting is present not only in milk allergy, but also in another ailment called *pyloric stenosis*. In pyloric stenosis, the valve that leads from the stomach to the duodenum is large and hypertonic, and it stops the free flow of milk between those two organs. A mother can diagnose the ailment of her baby by watching for certain symptoms. In allergy, vomiting starts immediately after birth, while in pyloric stenosis it starts a few weeks later. Also, in pyloric stenosis the vomiting is forceful, similar in effect to a projectile that lands at a distance from the baby. Lastly, pyloric stenosis is more frequently found in baby boys than girls, while milk allergy is found in both.

Even though the two main causes of vomiting in the early months of the atopic baby's life are milk allergy and pyloric stenosis, some other diseases may cause vomiting. These are described as follows.

Some babies regurgitate their milk with an audible belch after feeding. This may be caused by the ingestion of air from an empty bottle, or from a bottle that admits air through a faulty nipple, or because the baby takes his bottle too quickly and swallows air together with milk. Such regurgitation can be avoided by adjusting the size of the nipple, by removing the bottle before it is completely empty, and by handling the baby minimally after his feeding.

Vomiting may also be caused by undigested solid foods that are offered to the baby before he is able to chew them.

When the baby gets older, some of his vomiting may be "cyclic" or recurrent. This can be a manifestation of a childhood migraine occurring in high-strung children who have a gastrointestinal allergy as well.

Whether in the early months or later, acute infections and some abdominal conditions, such as intussusception, peritonitis, appendicitis, or incarcerated hernia, as well as diabetes, phenylketonuria, lead poisoning, injury to the head, epilepsy, or a brain tumor, may all cause vomiting.

Diarrhea

This is a condition of loose and watery stools caused by food contents moving through the digestive tract faster than normal. The result is insufficient time for proper water and nutrient absorption. In addition, a change in the color of the stools may occur because certain digestive juices have not had time to undergo the changes that normally occur.

A mother must recognize how normal stools look to recognize the abnormal ones. A baby may have three kinds of normal stools. The first discharge after birth is called *meconium*. It is made of secretions, bile, hair, and scalelike epithelial cells, usually semisolid. It has no odor and is greenish-brown. The baby has four to six emissions a day of this material for two to three days, and then goes on to have one of two other types of stool. If he is breastfed, the composition of the stools will be loose to pasty, normally not watery; their odor sour but not malodorous; their color medium to pale yellow, possibly green or light brown; the frequency two to four stools a day. If the child is fed cow's milk, the composition of the stools will be firmer and more homogeneous, the odor stronger and more malodorous, the color somewhat paler, the frequency less.

If the diarrhea is caused by allergy, eliminating milk from the diet will cause the diarrhea to stop. However, if the diarrhea is only one symptom among many, such as (1) a general or local infection caused either by viruses, bacteria, or protozoa; (2) a poisoning syndrome, caused either by a drug, by absorption of seeds found in fruits, by high-roughage food, or by an incompletely digested food given to the baby prematurely; (3) a general emotional disorder caused by fear and anxiety during a hospitalization, or a separation from parents; (4) an endocrine disease, such as hyperthyroidism; (5) a congenital deficiency, such as cystic fibrosis or celiac disease, then the treatment of the diarrhea would depend on eliminating its cause and neutralizing it.

Cystic fibrosis, incidentally, is a disease of the intestinal glands; it is usually associated with a chronic cough and severe hyponutrition. Celiac disease, on the other hand, is an ailment in which the intestines cannot properly digest the fats or the proteins (gluten) of wheat, rye, or barley. Clinically, a baby with cystic fibrosis or celiac disease looks sicker than a baby with milk allergy. Both of these ailments stunt his normal growth and make him appear older than he is, while milk allergy permits a baby to grow normally because he makes up for the lack of calories usually derived from milk by drinking fruit juices and eating other nutritious foods.

Treatment of Allergy to Milk

Milk is composed of butter, a sugar called *lactose,* and three different proteins, called *lactalbumin, B. lactoglobulin,* and *casein.* Boiling milk, or reducing it to powder through evaporation, may denature its two allergic proteins (B. lactoglobulin and lactalbumin) and make it harmless to the atopic baby. However, if using boiled or evaporated milk does not improve the allergic symptoms, and the baby continues to have diarrhea, colic, mucus in the stools, a stuffy nose, eczema, or asthma, then a substitute for milk must be considered. This is an important decision, one that has to be

ter first to give him a hypoallergenic cereal, such as rice, and
serve how he tolerates it. If he has no difficulty with it, a new
real can be added to his diet each week, leaving the addition of
orn to the very end because, being the most allergenic cereal, it
s one of the worst offenders among all the cereal grains. (Corn is
easily recognized as fresh or canned corn, cornmeal, breakfast
cereal, corn syrup, dextrose, corn oil or cornstarch. Corn oil is considered the least troublesome form of corn, while the most commonly offending form is corn syrup.)

Diagnosis

A baby who becomes suddenly cranky after the addition of a
cereal to his formula and suffers from vague and unexplained
symptoms, such as fatigue, irritability, loss of appetite, restlessness,
and so forth, or gets an outright allergic reaction such as colic,
vomiting, diarrhea, frequent colds, eczema, hives, or bronchial
asthma, should be suspected of being allergic to the cereal added
to his formula. Because skin tests for foods are most unreliable,
we must make use of an elimination diet to confirm the diagnosis.
The baby is put on a cereal-free diet for five days. If this gives
relief from symptoms, and if when the cereal is added again to the
diet the same symptoms recur, this is considered proof of allergy
to that cereal.

Treatment

Desensitization against cereals is not effective. The only way to
obtain relief from their symptoms is to eliminate them from the
diet for a period of three to four years. In this elimination, all cereal
grains are to be considered as members of one family, and are to
be removed from the diet of the baby who is allergic to any of them.
Poi is a good substitute for cereal grains. It is a Hawaiian food
derived from the taro root, and was introduced into baby feeding
by Dr. Jerome Glaser of Rochester, New York.

weighed carefully, for it involves depriving a baby not only of
milk, but of butter, cream, and cheese.

A good substitute for cow's milk is a formula prepared from the
plant of the soybean. Soybeans acquired importance in the nutrition of atopic babies in 1950. In that year, Dr. Jerome Glaser of
Rochester, New York, succeeded in raising many atopic babies who
were allergic to milk on extracts of soybean. Even though soybeans
were previously used to feed children, their high fat content did not
allow them to become a practical substitute for milk. A recent
discovery has permitted the separation of the fats from the proteins.
The new product has a new taste, a new texture, and a new look.
It is hypoallergenic and can be given with impunity to atopic children who suffer from multiple food allergies (milk and meat).

Besides acting as a substitute for milk and meats, the soybean
serves many other nutritional purposes. It is a source for cooking
and salad oils. Soybean flour, grits, and flakes are used in breads,
doughnuts, cakes, and cookies. Soybeans also serve as a splendid
emulsifier and binder in sausages and related meat products, in
breakfast foods, low-starch health foods, macaroni, noodles, con-
fections, and ice cream.

Soybeans have one great disadvantage: they have a bad taste.
The Chinese and the Indonesians will add a mold-based sauce to
them to make them not only palatable but a gourmet dish. The
sauce they add is, however, dangerous to children who are allergic
to molds. In America, the taste of soybeans is usually masked with
an extract of vanilla or honey.

Soybeans in the form of an equivalent to a milk-based formula
are sold under these names: Pro-Sobee, Mull Soy, Neo-Mull Soy,
Sobee, Soylac, Isomil. The form maintains the adequate nutritional
growth of a baby. It is high in unsaturated fats and therefore promotes easy digestion. Furthermore, it is white in color, has a
pleasant odor, a good vitamin and iron content, is sweet tasting,
promotes a physiologic stooling pattern, and is easily available.
Here is a breakdown of each of these products: *Isomil* (Ross) contains the soy isolate, together with sugar, unsaturated fat, corn,

coconut oil, vitamins, and iron. *Mull Soy* (Syntex) contains soy, unsaturated fat, sugar, vitamins, and iron. *Neo-Mull Soy* (Syntex) contains soy and a supplement of an important amino acid (methionine) to increase its biological value, plus vitamins and iron. *Pro-Sobee* (Mead-Johnson) contains soy, unsaturated fat, coconut oil, sugar, maltose, dextrins, vitamins, and iron. *Sobee* (Mead-Johnson) contains soy, unsaturated fat, coconut oil, sugar, maltose, dextrins, vitamins, and iron. *Soylac* (Loma Linda) contains soy, sugar maltose, dextrins, vitamins, and iron.

In choosing the right food for a baby, the pediatrician has to adapt a soy formula suitable to the needs of the baby.

The babies who do not tolerate soybeans have to be fed Nutramigen or minced lamb instead. Dr. Albert Rowe has elaborated a formula based on strained lamb, a formula that is a complete and healthful diet.

Rowe's Strained Lamb Formula

2 tablespoons potato flour or 2½ tablespoons tapioca flour
½ teaspoon salt
1 teaspoon calcium carbonate
2 tablespoons sugar
4 cups water, approximately
8 ounces strained lamb (available in jars)
3½ tablespoons sesame oil or soy oil

Combine the flour, salt, calcium carbonate, and sugar in 1 cup of water. Cook over low heat for 10 minutes, then add the meat, oil, and enough water to make a volume of 4½ cups. Cook over low heat for 10 minutes more.
Note: Reduce the amount of flour if you wish a thinner product.

A Case History
Subject: X.L. (male)
Age: 2 months
Symptoms: X.L. was born to allergic parents. He did not take to his
    formula and did not thrive on it. He vomited frequently, had
    diarrhea, often had gas, and had canker sores in his mouth.

Diagnosis and treatment: His general practitio
    milk and put him on soybean milk. He t
    gained weight, stopped vomiting, and had
    examined once every four weeks for weight, l
    ference, and blood chemistries. All the results w
    limits. The soy formula provided this baby with
    looked like milk, poured like milk, had a pleasa.
    milky sweet taste. The change was acceptable no
    mother, but to the allergic baby, who did not develo
    allergies, as well.

The Addition of Solid Foods to the Diet

An atopic baby should have a solid food added to his diet at
months of age. By then his alimentary tract will have matured, a
will not easily absorb incompletely digested food, which is sensi
tizing. We must keep in mind that a baby who consumes adequate
calories in the formula, takes in all the essential nutrients, and gets
a reasonable distribution in his diet of protein, fat, and carbohydrates, does not necessarily require solids in his diet. We add the
solids, however, because they do offer some advantages. They
provide essential foods that may not be present in adequate amount
in the formula; they help balance the calories derived from proteins,
fats, and carbohydrates; and they adjust the baby's caloric intake
to a desirable level.

Allergy to Cereals

In America the first solid food added to the formula is usually a
mixture of various cereal grains.

By "cereals" is meant wheat, rice, barley, rye, corn, and malt.
All baby cereals come partially cooked and ready to use, either in
a pure form or as mixtures. It is not wise to force a baby into eating
cereals. It will take him two to three weeks to really adjust to them,
and his initial refusal may or may not be a sign of allergy.

An atopic baby should not be started on mixed cereals. It is

Allergy to Other Foods

Fruit

Fruit is usually the second solid food added to the diet. However, in countries that have an abundance of citrus fruits, like Israel, the first solid food is the orange. Fresh orange juice is usually well tolerated, but because it is highly allergenic it should not be given to an atopic baby until he is five months old; the juice is first frozen and then diluted with water because freezing, canning, and dilution make the juice less allergenic. If the baby tolerates orange juice in this form, it can be followed by fresh orange juice.

Apples, peaches, prunes, apricots, or pears can similarly be added to the diet, but must be stewed first. Berries—strawberries, raspberries, and so forth—frequently cause hives, abdominal discomfort, or throat irritation, and therefore should not be eaten at all by the atopic baby. If the baby is allergic to fruits in general, he must take ascorbic acid (vitamin C) daily.

Vegetables

Vegetables—fresh, frozen, boiled, and strained or pureed—may be added to the diet three weeks after fruit. These are available ready made in jars; they can also be ground up in large quantities. In general, they do not cause allergies; further, squash, string beans, peas, carrots, beets, and sweet potatoes are less allergenic than tomatoes, onions, or cabbage. Spinach contains histamine, gives many false positive reactions on testing, and is to be avoided since it may cause chapping of the lips and anus.

Eggs

Egg allergy is a severe and dangerous illness. It is very hard to outgrow, and may persist for many years. It may be so severe that just touching or smelling an egg may cause a reaction.

In order to reduce the chances of an allergic reaction to egg (a highly allergenic but extremely important food to a baby because of its iron content), some precautions must be taken. Egg may be added to the diet at one year of age and not earlier; it must be thoroughly cooked in order to reduce its allergenic powers; its white part must be removed after cooking, and only the hard-boiled yolk given; it must be tried in very small amounts initially.

Allergy to egg usually manifests itself as an itch, hives, or eczema, and its sole treatment consists in removing all eggs— chicken, duck, turkey, or those of any other fowl—from the diet. But this treatment will not be effective unless it is complete. Even the plates and spoons of the child must be of a disposable nature to avoid previous contamination by eggs.

An egg-sensitive baby should not be vaccinated against flu, German measles, or mumps—as all these vaccines are egg cultures of a virus. If vaccination is imperative, the special precautions listed later on in this chapter must be observed.

Meats

Meats, either fresh or canned, are to be introduced into the baby's diet at six months. Beef, lamb, or pork can be used. Lamb is the least, while pork is the most, allergenic meat. All parts of the animal—such as the liver, kidneys, sweetbreads, or brains—can be given to the baby.

Fish

Fish are highly allergenic foods, even though canned fish is better tolerated than fresh fish. Fish can be boiled or broiled, and fed to the baby at about one year of age. If the baby has already shown multiple food allergies, it is better to forget about fish altogether and stick to lamb as a source of protein in the baby's diet.

Shellfish

Shellfish—such as crab, lobster, oysters, shrimp, scallops, mussels, abalone, clams, squid, and crayfish—are all extremely dangerous foods and should never be given to the atopic baby.

Beverages

Those, besides milk and fruit juices, that are frequently given to children include tea, coffee, chocolate, cola, ginger ale, and other soft drinks. Tea is the safest of them all, and can be given in moderate quantities to a child, especially when he has diarrhea.

Chocolate

Chocolate is derived from the cocoa bean, and simultaneous allergy to its relative, the cola drink, is common. Since such a large

Comparative Feeding Schedules of a Nonallergic Baby and a Potentially Allergic Baby

Age	Nonallergic	Potentially Allergic
1 month	If breastfed, add water and orange juice	Add water only
2 months	Add iron, extra vitamin A, D, and C	Same
4 months	Add cereals, vegetables, fruits	Add rice only
6 months	Give whole milk, egg yolk, meats, and fish	Give orange juice and lamb
8 months	Give regular foods, all mashed	Add vegetables
10 months	Start to limit milk intake	Add beef and pork
12 months	Give regular food	Add egg yolk and fish
2 years	Encourage self-feeding	Add beverages and encourage self-feeding

number of foods—candies, cakes, cookies, drinks, ice cream, syrups, and pies—may contain chocolate, this explains the frequency with which the allergic symptoms of chocolate—sneezing, wheezing, hives, eczema, nasal stuffiness, coughing, headache, gastrointestinal pain, gas, diarrhea, fatigue, nasal polyps, and dizziness—are found. However, even though these symptoms are frequently encountered in allergy to chocolate, they are not specific to chocolate, and may denote an allergy to another type of food.

Cara Coa is an adequate substitute for chocolate. It is derived from the carob tree, and its taste is like that of chocolate.

PREVENTING AND DIAGNOSING FOOD ALLERGIES

An atopic baby should be breastfed as much as possible, and as long as possible. If the baby cannot be breastfed, he must take a formula that provides twenty calories per ounce and consume two and one-half to three ounces of the formula per pound of body weight. There is no advantage in adding allergenic foods to his diet early; these should be added in this fashion: fresh juices at six months of age, egg in the later months of the first year, fish in the first year; shellfish, nuts, mustard, peanut butter, and berries are not to be given at all.

A child with migraine headaches, hives, perennial clogging of the nose, eczema, or asthma, who vomits often, does not eat well, has diarrhea, and dislikes certain specific foods, should be suspected of suffering from a food allergy. Such a baby should be kept on a hypoallergenic diet that consists of tea, Ry Krisp, rice, olive oil, lamb, any vegetable, ripe olives, and Jell-O, with no fresh fruit, milk, fish or shellfish, nuts, or chocolate, and be observed for one week. If he improves, he is probably allergic to one or more foods and he should be brought to a pediatric allergist for an exact diagnosis. This can be a difficult job because there are many shortcomings, listed below, in the diagnostic methods we use to detect food allergies.

1. Food histories are unreliable because an allergy to a food

manifests itself two to three days after the food is eaten, and its symptoms may be so mild as to go unnoticed. The only exceptions to this rule are the severe reactions to infrequently eaten foods.

2. Intracutaneous testing for foods, a practice that is full of possible errors.

3. Elimination diets and the deliberate feeding of suspected foods, both of which have many pitfalls because there are many ways in which a small quantity of a food may be introduced unknowingly to a diet. Example: two kinds of foods may have been cooked at different times in the same container, which was in the meantime not washed, or an allergenic food may have been wrapped in plastic and then that wrapper used to wrap a nonallergenic food.

4. An exacerbation of symptoms in food allergies may be caused by nonspecific triggering factors, such as chilling, exertion, infection, additives, inhalants, chemicals, and drugs.

5. The fact that a food allergy is different from a gastrointestinal allergy. Food allergy is expressed by vomiting, gas, diarrhea, asthma, rhinitis, or eczema; while gastrointestinal allergy, even though similarly expressed by vomiting, gas, or diarrhea, may be caused not only by allergy to a food, but also by allergy to inhalants and injectants as well.

6. A summation effect may complicate a food allergy. Two foods which cause no trouble when each one is given alone may cause trouble when both are given at the same time. Likewise, a synergistic effect between a food and an inhalant may exist, such as an intolerance of melons and bananas only during the ragweed season.

Conclusion: It is hard to diagnose a food allergy because of many potential errors.

EFFECT OF FOOD ALLERGY ON GROWTH AND DEVELOPMENT

The most common cause of poor growth in a baby is improper nutrition. A baby with food allergies who has to have many essential amino acids or other nutrients eliminated from his regular diet may not develop normally. The mother of the baby and the baby's doctor must compare his development with that of a normal baby and decide whether the baby is doing well or not.

During the first month, a baby's hearing is well developed, but his eyes may appear crossed. He yawns, hiccups, sneezes, and sleeps all the time, except when being fed.

In the second month he starts to settle into a regular routine of sleeping through the night, and can turn his head in the direction of voices.

In the third month he smiles, holds up his head, and enjoys bright colors.

In the fourth month he holds up his head and can grasp a toy.

In the fifth month he doubles his birth weight, carries everything to his mouth, and wants to be lifted.

In the sixth month he can sit and show emotion; his first teeth appear.

In the seventh month he starts crawling and calls "mama" and "dada."

In the ninth to twelfth months, he crawls, stands without support, says a few words, has six to eight teeth, and weighs in at triple his birth weight. A well-nourished baby will double the length he was at two years by the time he reaches eighteen.

The following are three case histories of children who were allergic to foods.

A Case History: Multiple Food Allergy

Subject: S.J. (male)

Age: 3 months

Symptoms: Bloating, vomiting, diarrhea, canker sores, aphthous ulcers, inflamed tongue since birth.

Diagnosis: A pediatrician suggested allergy to milk.

Treatment: The pediatrician prescribed boiling the formula and then refrigerating it before use. After two weeks the child did not improve, and he was put on goat's milk. With that, the child improved slightly. As cereals were added to the child's diet, the symptoms increased to include a rash, stuffed nose, and stool with a bad odor.

The child was then seen by an allergist, who tested him for allergy to milk and cereal grains. He uncovered a marked reaction to corn and a negative one to milk. Even then, his clinical diagnosis was allergy to milk as well as to corn. He advised that all milk products as well as cereal grains be removed from S.J.'s diet. A week later, all symptoms disappeared. The cereals were then reinstated in the diet, successively, one every ten days; only when corn was added did the symptoms return. The allergist then advised S.J.'s mother that her son would have to avoid corn for many years and milk for one more year, and to consult him again then.

Note: Allergy to foods has to be diagnosed clinically, as we have previously mentioned, because skin tests are not as conclusive in food allergy as they are in inhalant allergy. That is why the allergist removed milk as well as corn from the diet, even though the child had a negative skin reaction to milk.

A Case History: Hives Caused by Chocolate

Subject: J.A.

Age: 1 year

Symptoms: Hives. On Christmas Day, J.A. was fed a piece of chocolate for the first time in her life. Several hours later, she suffered an attack of giant hives.

Diagnosis and Treatment: Clinical allergy to chocolate. However, a general practitioner performed eighty-seven scratch tests on J.A. and prepared a mixture for desensitization. The injections made her sick each time she took them, but the hives did not return.

Comments: The diagnosis was right, but the treatment wrong. J.A. should never have been skin tested, as the cause of the hives was self-evident—the chocolate. The fact that J.A. showed a positive reaction to allergens did not mean that she was clinically allergic to those substances.

Desensitization against potential allergens is a costly procedure that does not prevent the development of allergies. J.A. should merely have eliminated chocolate from her diet.

A Case History: Allergy to Pork

Subject: J.B.

Age: 1 year

Current complaint: Persistent pain in abdomen and bronchial asthma.

Family history: Father is asthmatic; mother has hay fever.

Personal History: The child vomited once every four to five days and was very sensitive to the touch of his upper abdomen. The pains were severe enough to warrant X rays of the stomach, but the examinations were negative. Furthermore, the child looked pale and tired and suffered from frequent colds. At times he had asthma, which did not respond to antibiotics.

Diagnosis: An allergist suspected a food allergy and performed skin tests for foods. They turned out to be negative. An elimination diet pointed to pork.

Treatment: J.B. was made to avoid pork. Ten days after this type of diet was instituted, he had no abdominal pain, no asthma, and felt in general better. Two years later he was still free of symptoms.

Comments: Even though pork is not usually fed to a one-year-old baby, the doctor took it into consideration in the elimination diet.

Although the mother's main concern was the pain in the abdomen, that pain was really a secondary symptom in the food allergy syndrome that was causing the bronchial asthma.

IMMUNIZATIONS AND THE ATOPIC BABY

Kinds of Immunization

An atopic child needs to be immunized against diphtheria, whooping cough, tetanus, measles, German measles, mumps, and polio.

Timetable for Immunization

A visit to a pediatrician's office once a month is a must for an atopic baby. The pediatrician will check the baby's diet, growth, and general well-being, and at the same time give him his inoculations. It is a good idea to write down the dates of all the baby's immunizations and his allergies because this information is very valuable if the baby goes on a trip or if he changes pediatricians. The Committee of Infectious Diseases of the American Academy of Pediatrics in 1971 gave the following schedule of immunizations:

1. At two months, four months, and six months, DPT vaccine and trivalent oral polio. At eighteen months and five years, a booster dose of each. At twelve months, measles vaccine. At two years, rubella and mumps vaccines. At fifteen years, combined tetanus and diphtheria toxoids (TD).

2. Tetanus toxoid should be given at the time of injury. For clean minor wounds, no booster dose is needed by a fully immunized child unless more than ten years have elapsed since the last dose. For contaminated wounds, a booster dose should be given if more than five years have elapsed since the last dose.

3. Smallpox vaccination is not required now as a routine procedure, because in the United States the risk of catching smallpox is now less than the risk of a severe reaction to the vaccine.

Latest Immunization Requirements for Children Entering School

The following immunizations are now required by the New York schools, unless there is a religious objection or a medical reason why the child cannot receive the shots.

Measles

Each child must have one dose of live measles vaccine. The injection would, of course, not have to be administered if the child has recovered from measles contracted naturally.

Rubella

The state requires one dose of live rubella vaccine for children up to eleven years of age.

Poliomyelitis

Either five doses of Salk vaccine must be given, or doses of an oral vaccine. If the oral vaccine is administered, it should be one dose each of monovalent oral vaccine (types 1, 3, and 2) plus one dose of trivalent. An alternative would be three doses of trivalent oral vaccine.

Diphtheria

A primary series of three injections is required for each child, followed by a booster.

General Rules for Immunizations

1. No immunization of any kind is to be given to an atopic baby unless he looks and feels healthy.

2. While giving an immunizing injection, a doctor should keep on hand a vial of adrenalin for possible allergic reactions.

3. Inoculations against diphtheria, pertussis, and tetanus are usually given together. Such a vaccination is called DPT. It may cause fever, crankiness, loss of appetite, and soreness around the injection site. These reactions disappear after twenty-four hours and require only baby aspirin for treatment. At times, DPT may cause a severe local reaction, as well as a high temperature. If that happens, the next injection of DPT should be broken down into its single components and each component should be given individually on a future date. Also, a child who has suffered a severe reaction from DPT should not get any other mixed immunization, such as MMR, but rather should get separate injections for measles, mumps, and rubella.

4. A smallpox vaccination, when mandatory, should be deferred in an atopic baby who is prone to skin rashes as long as possible (one or two years). When it is done, the mother should take special care of the vaccination site. This must be left uncovered for twenty-

four hours until it dries up completely. Following this, it may be sponge washed until the third or fourth day. If the vaccination "takes," a red pimple appears on the fourth day. By the sixth day the pimple appears bigger, is more tender, itches, and contains pus. By the eighth day it develops a crust or a scale, which remains until the twelfth day and then falls off. The whole process should be complete within a period of two or three weeks. Smallpox vaccination should not be given in summer, or when the child or a member of his family has eczema. If vaccination is imperative in a child with eczema, then the method advised by Dr. Henry Kempe of Colorado should be used. The material of the Kempe vaccine is available only in special institutions.

Smallpox vaccination was performed for the first time by Edward Jenner in 1796. Using vaccine obtained from a milkmaid who had contracted cowpox, a mild disease, he provided immunity to a young boy against the dreaded smallpox.

5. Sabin vaccine is an oral polio virus vaccine. It is an attenuated live vaccine that is safe, yet gives long-lasting immunity against polio.

6. Egg-sensitive children may not tolerate the flu vaccination because the vaccine may contain egg. A skin test with the vaccine must precede its administration. There is a controversy on the value of this vaccination, and it must not be given indiscriminately to all atopic children. If the skin test is negative, the vaccine is to be given only to asthma-prone children who are five years or more, and only in time of epidemics. When given, it should be done in this manner: 0.1 cc. of the vaccine is to be given intracutaneously, to be repeated in two weeks and again in two months. Because the intracutaneous administration causes sloughing of the skin, some allergists prefer to give it subcutaneously instead. The vaccine used should be free from alum, be polyvalent, and contain the suspected virus. If the skin test is positive, then that child should avoid not only the flu vaccine, but the mumps, measles, or rubella vaccines as well, because all of these vaccines may contain egg. However, not a single anaphylactic reaction has been described after the use

of these vaccines in egg-sensitive children, even though theoretically this may happen.

Benefits of Immunization and Problems for the Future

Now that polio, measles, and smallpox have ceased to be major problems in the United States because of early vaccination, mumps and rubella will probably follow suit, as will serum sickness, because human serum has replaced horse serum in this country in the preparation of antitoxins. This, however, is not what is happening in the rest of the world. Millions in Asia and Africa will continue to have these diseases for years to come because they lack medical facilities. Because of increased air travel, many people from these areas are visiting the United States. We can expect that some of them will bring along problems connected with these diseases, problems that may represent further difficulties for the doctors of the United States for many years in the future.

Vaccination Doldrums

Even though smallpox vaccination has now ceased to be mandatory, there is no reason to neglect any other kind of vaccination through indifference, neglect, or ignorance. This can be disastrous to the child as well as to his community. Medical care is dispensed free of charge by many sources, such as practicing physicians, community clinics, schools, outpatient clinics, and health department clinics. These are ready at any time to give vaccinations to any child, no matter what his financial status, who may be in need of them.

Other Recommended Immunizations

Although immunizations against whooping cough and tetanus are not legally required, the Department of Health recommends that a basic series of shots be administered to a child, followed by a booster dose within two years of school entry. A tuberculin test should also be given to children in the twelfth grade.

If the dosages given the atopic child are different from those mentioned above and the doctor feels they are adequate, it will be necessary for him to provide a statement saying that in his opinion the child is adequately protected against the diseases without any further follow-up.

In any case, once the child has been immunized, the law requires that the doctor provide the parents with a certification showing that he has fulfilled the state requirement. In addition to immunization, a physical examination is mandatory for all children entering school.

Serum Sickness

A child who does not get his basic immunization against tetanus has to have an injection of horse serum containing ready-made antibodies against tetanus each time he gets a cut. Serum sickness is an allergic reaction to this injection. Its symptoms are hives, swelling of the joints and fever. It occurs in 10 percent of allergic children if 10 cc. of serum are injected; its incidence goes up to 90 percent if 100 cc. are injected. The reaction is either immediate (minutes after the injection), delayed (hours after the injection), or accelerated (days after the injection).

In case a child has to be given antitetanus horse serum and he is known to be allergic to horse serum, then a human serum rich in tetanus antibodies should be used instead. This serum is available commercially.

A Case History: Serum Sickness
Subject: M.N.
Age: 8 years
History and Symptoms: M.N. was a Chinese (Hong Kong) girl who
    came to the United States without having ever had her basic

immunizations. While in this country, she developed a large dirty cut while gardening. A doctor injected her with a tetanus-immune horse serum and a tetanus toxoid. The serum was meant to protect her immediately against tetanus, and the toxoid to give her long-range immunity against it. Fifteen minutes after the injections, M.N. became pale and dizzy, and she collapsed. She was revived with an adrenalin injection. Eight days later she developed fever, hives, and pains in the joints. This was diagnosed as serum sickness and treated with antihistamines.

Complication: One week later, M.N. complained of constant headache, low-grade temperature, vomiting, and a red-colored urine. The doctor admitted her to the hospital with a diagnosis of nephritis (a kidney ailment).

Comments: M.N.'s treatment was correct—the antitetanic horse serum was administered rightly in order to prevent tetanus then and there, and the toxoid was rightly given in order to give her immunity against a future tetanus infection. A known calculated risk of a possible reaction to the serum injection was taken. This led to a rare complication in the kidneys.

M.N. should have had her tetanus immunizations in China before she entered the United States. A tetanus toxoid booster would have been sufficient to treat the cut, and she would not have needed the horse serum that gave her the nephritis.

M.N. was eight years old when she became sick with serum sickness. Serum sickness, however, can occur at any age. This case history is being used to illustrate an unnecessary complication from a badly carried out immunization program that pertains to the first year.

Anaphylaxis

An injection of horse serum, penicillin, or a desensitizing serum may sometimes cause an allergic reaction far more dangerous than serum sickness. Such a reaction is called *anaphylactic shock,* and it may endanger the life of a child unless it is treated immediately. Shock itself is a condition in which the capillaries become so paralyzed that their perfusion is inadequate to sustain life. In shock, the vital cells starve for oxygen and their metabolic products remain in them because of poor circulation. It is an emergency situation that has to be dealt with immediately; otherwise, cellular injury may result. This can progress to organ failure and death. In anaphylactic shock, the blood serum leaks out of the capillaries into the connective tissue, the mucus secretion of the glands of the lung mucosa increases, and there is a spasm of the smooth muscles of the bronchi. These changes bring about the following symptoms: hives, a congestion in the nose and eyes, wheezing and asthma, low blood pressure, and swelling in many parts of the body. Anaphylactic shock may also be caused by drugs taken orally or by allergy to a food.

Because the risks of anaphylactic shock are so great, any injection of horse serum, penicillin, or desensitizing material should be avoided unless it is absolutely necessary. Here is a summary of the causes, the allergic tests, and the treatment of anaphylaxis:

The principal offenders are drugs such as penicillin, aspirin, ACTH, venom of bees and insects, and injected allergens. Penicillin allergy is usually preceded by a local or systemic reaction; aspirin allergy has a history of asthma and nasal polyps; allergy to the venom of bees and other insects has a history of an ever-increasing local reaction, and the same goes for injected allergens.

The allergic tests for these offenders are not conclusive, especially in the case of penicillin and aspirin. However, with injected allergens and bee stings, intracutaneous tests are helpful.

The treatment of allergy to penicillin, aspirin, and ACTH through desensitization is not recommended. It is highly successful in bee and insect allergens.

NOTE TO THE GENERAL PRACTITIONER

For any general practitioner who may be using this book, here is some information detailing what an emergency kit for a doctor to counter anaphylactic shock should contain: adrenalin 1:1000 (in a multiple-dose vial), aminophylline (two ampoules of 250 mg.), glucose 5 percent in distilled water (250 cc.), an injectable antihistamine preparation, endotracheal tubes (child size), one tracheotomy set, one tourniquet, an oxygen tank and mask resuscitator, needles and syringes as needed.

ECZEMAS

These are a number of varied skin ailments frequent among babies. They are all characterized by the presence of rashes, redness, swelling, weeping, fissuring, scaling, and itching in different areas of the body.

History of Baby Eczemas

Four thousand years ago, Chinese doctors knew that eczema was caused by intolerance to foods. Two thousand years later, Hippocrates connected hives to a stomach disturbance; Bateman remarked on the frequency with which urticaria was produced by shellfish; Quincke and Osler mentioned a hereditary factor in urticaria. In more recent times, Ramazzini studied children whose skin was predisposed to eczema; Jadassohn discovered the patch test for contact eczema that Sulzberger popularized in America; and recently Ishizaka discovered that the amount of IgE present in the serum of a baby with eczema is directly related to the gravity of his condition.

Prevention

Babies have a delicate skin. It can be easily irritated by the bleaches and detergents used in cleaning diapers, an irritation that can bring about infection and eczema.

To prevent this:

1. Use no bleaches or detergents to clean the clothing or the diapers of the baby.

2. Apply unscented baby oil to the skin of the baby once a day if it appears dry.

3. Use talcum powder on the skin of the baby after baths to dry it.

Diaper Rash

This is an irritation of the skin under the diapers caused by prolonged contact of the skin with urine and feces. Almost all babies develop it, despite every possible care simply because they cannot be toilet trained at an early age.

The condition comes about in the following manner. Bacteria migrate from the rectum to the soaked diapers. They break up the urea found in them into ammonia. Ammonia then irritates the skin of the buttocks, macerates it, and exposes it to infection. The prevention of diaper rash can be achieved with:

1. Cleanliness of the child's whole body by means of daily bathing.

2. Avoidance of wet diapers, which moisten the skin.

3. Avoidance of soiled diapers to prevent infection.

4. Avoidance of bleaches and detergents in cleaning the diapers because these may cause chafing and soreness in the diaper area. Proper care of diapers should be achieved by rinsing the soiled diapers in the toilet bowl immediately after changing the baby, keeping them in a covered diaper pail containing water before washing them, and storing them in a clean covered container. Furthermore, the diapers should be *boiled* once every two to three days to kill ammonia-forming bacteria. Washing is not enough to kill such bacteria.

5. Avoidance of low water intake, because this makes the urine concentrated and acidy.

6. Avoidance of loose bowels, which irritate the skin around the anus and buttocks.

When diarrhea is present, it is best to use disposable diapers and change them often. Whenever possible, one must avoid plastic or rubber pants over the diapers. They are convenient, but they seal in both heat and moisture; this increases the possibility of irritation, while the elastic bands around the legs cause abrasions.

After the soiled diaper is removed, the diaper area should be sponged with warm water and gently dried with a soft towel, special attention being paid to the skin folds. The area should then be sprinkled with a baby powder or plain talc.

In the summer, the baby should not be dressed over the diaper area, as this may lead to prickly heat and diaper rash. He should only wear a sleeveless shirt besides his diapers. Furthermore, he should be exposed to the air and sun in moderation and without risking irritation or a sunburn.

The treatment of diaper rash consists of saline dressing or Burow's solution (1:100 with tap water), which should be applied to the inflamed area for fifteen to thirty minutes twice daily. This is to be followed by an application of a bland paste, such as zinc ointment. If the rash is infected with a fungus called *monilia,* then nystatin ointment is more efficacious than zinc ointment. If the infection keeps recurring and causes a thickening of the skin, it needs a vioform-cortisone ointment. If none of the above methods of treatment work, the baby has to be left unclothed, in a properly heated room, for a few days.

There is a skin irritation called *intertrigo,* which may look similar to a diaper rash. It is a laceration of the skin between the buttocks of overweight children brought about by the rubbing of the buttocks against each other and the sweating in that area during the hot summer months. To treat this condition, the laceration has to be covered, in between the buttocks, with a soft gauze, over which may be sprinkled some Neosporin powder to control the infection.

Cradle Cap or Seborrheic Dermatitis

This condition, a nuisance rather than a disease, is the most prevalent form of eczema in babies and children. It is simply a normal process of scaling that has gone to extremes. The condition manifests itself as an inflamed, red, greasy, and scaly area that appears over the scalp, eyebrows, or chest and that becomes irritated when washed with soap and water. While its spontaneous recovery is possible, it is not frequent. Its treatment consists of cleansing the area with baby oil twice daily; severe cases may need a medicated shampoo or a hydrocortisone ointment. Sometimes the condition is associated with emotional lability, and older children may benefit from mild tranquilization.

Atopic Dermatitis or Eczema

This is an important skin disorder of atopic babies. Although we do not know its cause, we do know that the child who has eczema has an irritable skin that is easily influenced by allergic, psychogenic, climatic, or environmental factors. Specifically, these factors are changes in environmental temperature, irritating clothing (wool, silk, rayon), irritating soaps and detergents, allergies to foods and inhalants, emotional stress, physical exercise and sweating, infections, tight clothing, or greasy occlusive ointments. Among all the allergenic causes of eczema, cow's milk, egg, and wheat are the most frequent; however, the results of skin tests to these foods are often negative, and the improvement after the elimination of these foods from the diet is the only clue to their being a cause of the ailment.

Children with atopic eczema are more likely than normal children to develop hay fever and asthma later on in life.

Clinical Picture of Atopic Eczema

1. Eczema begins at any age, but more frequently in the first months of life. It may improve during childhood, disappear, appear again at puberty, and persist into middle life.

2. The rash of eczema is itchy and has a predilection to certain areas of the body: cheeks, wrists, elbows, neck, chest, and backs of the knees.

3. The frequently scratched eczematous skin gets excoriations, oozing, crusting, thickening, inflammation, a change of color from white to dark, and the hair falls off.

4. An eczematous child who scratches all night, and therefore does not sleep well, inevitably suffers from chronic fatigue.

To Diagnose an Atopic Eczema, We Need:

1. The appearance of an itchy rash in early infancy.
2. An association of this rash with hay fever or asthma, or a food allergy.
3. A family history of atopy.

Complications

1. Infections: (a) Bacterial infections may occur in the scratched fissures; and (b) viral infections may occur from a dissemination of a simple herpex or a smallpox vaccination. These two viral infections are extremely dangerous complications of eczemas. Smallpox dissemination can be avoided by skipping vaccination altogether, and also by avoiding contact with siblings who have been vaccinated recently.
2. Emotional involvement caused by sleepless nights.
3. Allergic sensitization and anaphylaxis from the use of allergenic drugs.

The "Management" of Atopic Eczema

This subject should be approached with guarded enthusiasm, as there is no way to "cure" an eczema, any more than one can cure diabetes. Its goals should be limited to an alleviation of the discomfort of the itch, and an improvement of the aesthetics of the skin. To achieve these two purposes, we use applications of lotions, creams, and ointments.

A lotion, which has to be shaken before it can be used, is a powder suspended in water. When the water evaporates, the powder is left on the eczema. An ointment is a medicine put in a fat of animal or vegetable origin. Its purpose is to soften the upper layer of the skin so that the medicine can penetrate the inner layers. A cream is a fat that can hold water as well as a medicine.

We need all of these vehicles to bring a medicine to the skin because the treatment of baby eczema does not depend on its cause but on the actual changes it brings about in the skin structure. Also, in treating eczema we have to keep in mind that eczema needs an element of time to heal, as well as a respect for the integrity of the skin.

Acutely inflamed eczema subsides with continuous or intermittent applications of normal saline. Gauze, old diapers, or old cotton shirts can be used for the compresses, which have to be removed every two to three hours and remoistened. Their temperature may vary from extremely cold compresses for localized eruptions, swellings, or hives, to extremely hot compresses in pruritic rashes. Subacute inflammations need either lotions or creams, depending on how moist or dry the skin may be, and chronic inflammations need ointments or tapes to soften the hardened skin. Extensive inflammations that cover many parts of the body need baths.

These general principles need to be illustrated.

If the eczema is minimal and its area is small, a few local wet dressings of a normal saline solution (2 teaspoons salt per quart of water), or plain milk or a milk solution (4 quarts of milk to 1 quart water) may be enough.

If the eczema is minimal but the affected area is extensive, then a medicated bath has to be used, such as a starch bath, which consists of one cup Aveeno per tub, or a bran bath, which is one pound of bran in a cheesecloth bag per tub.

If the eczema is minimal in intensity and area, but infected, soaking it with a towel wet with Burow's solution (1:100 with tap water) or Domeboro powder (1 packet or 1 tablet per pint of tap water) should be enough.

However, if the skin area is *minimal,* but *very infected,* an antibiotic-containing ointment, such as Neosporin ointment, may be needed. If the infection is caused by a fungus called *monilia,* either Whitefield's tincture lotion, Fungizone lotion, Mycolog ointment, or Myocostatin should be used.

If the eczema consists of a small localized rash over normal skin, either a hydrocortisone ointment (Kenalog, Cordran), a cortisone spray (Deca-Spray), or a cortisone tape can be applied. Medicated cortisone tape is easily applied. Not bulky, it is also transparent, slightly elastic, very flexible, moisture proof, and contains corticosteroids in its adhesive part. It is three inches wide and is supplied in rolls up to eighty inches long. It is anti-inflammatory, antipruritic and vasoconstrictive, and may be left on the skin for twelve hours at a time. It is recommended for adjunctive treatment of dry skin, scaling, and localized lesions of atopic dermatitis. It is, however, relatively three times as costly as cortisone in a jar or tube.

If the eczema happens to be on a dry skin, an emollient bath, such as Alpha Keri, Aveen-Oil, Mellobath, or Geri-Bath (1 or 2 teaspoons per tub) should be used. If that same rash has become chronic and the skin has hardened, tar baths, such as Zetar emulsion, Balnetar, Junitar Bath, or Ar-Exbath (1 to 2 teaspoons per tub), work best.

The use of steroids incorporated in a vehicle on skin infected with eczema has revolutionized its treatment. Their dosage comes in full strength, half strength or quarter strength, depending on the amount of active ingredient incorporated in the vehicle. The vehicle of the steroid is extremely important, and it should vary with the type of skin on which it is used. If the eczema is on a hairy skin, the vehicle must be a nonwashable ointment; if it is in a skin fold that is moist, a lotion would work better; if it is on a dry skin, a water-washable cream does best; and for certain inaccessible areas, sprays may give better results.

Prolonged application of hormones on the skin may cause skin atrophy, systemic absorption of the hormones, and allergy to the vehicle that carries the hormones.

In case systemic absorption is suspected, one has to check for infections, ulcers, diabetes, osteoporosis, hypertension, glaucoma, and cataract. A periodic examination including blood pressure, a chest X ray, blood count, urinalysis, a stool exam for blood, and checkups for fractures, have to be performed regularly. Prolonged use of the hormones may also cause a retention of sodium and water, giving rise to a moon-face, and the loss of muscle tone.

Hospitalization and Eczema

At times, some refractory cases of eczema do better when hospitalized, because in the hospital babies with such cases of eczema are removed from their usual environment, with its attendant physical and emotional stresses. Furthermore, they can be better sedated, and their topical treatment can be controlled more easily.

Contact Dermatitis

All baby eczemas appear during the first year. However, some forms of contact dermatitis occur later. These are (1) hand eczema and (2) eczema caused by clothing. We put them here for convenience.

Hand Eczema

This is an eczema that occurs in school-age children. It follows a prolonged contact with soaps, detergents, and many chemicals a child may handle in his schoolwork, hobbies, or just in the course of his everyday living, such as paints, glues, insect repellents, fruit juices, bleaches, perfumes, deodorants, dyes, and sprays.

Hand eczema manifests itself as tiny, watery blisters on the sides of the fingers. If the blisters are scratched open, a raw, oozing area, which is inflamed and painful, appears. If the blisters remain closed, they become dry and scaly. In both cases, the skin eventually heals and returns to normal in a period of a week. Meanwhile, new blisters may appear on the other parts of the same hand or on the other hand. These blisters may either disappear altogether or may keep recurring at irregular intervals.

The name "hand eczema" is related to its place on the hand of the child, and not to its cause. Its cause is either an allergy to one of the above-mentioned agents, or an irritation caused by a prolonged contact with that agent.

Prevention of contact eczema consists of (1) wearing two pairs of gloves when working with liquid irritants—that is, a pair of cotton gloves under a pair of rubber gloves with a rubber band at the wrist (lined gloves are not sufficient) or (2) using a silicone cream. Silicote and Siliconex may be used to cover the hand, but a 30 to 40 percent concentration of silicone is needed in those creams so that they become effective insulating agents.

Treatment is the same as for any other kind of eczema. It consists of local baths, wet dressings, application of lotions and cortisone tape, tranquilizers by mouth.

Eczema Caused by Clothing

Because clothing is in intimate contact with the skin of a child it may cause eczemas. Some of these eczemas are merely irritations caused by friction, while others are due to an allergy. Leather, wool, mohair, rayon, nylon, and many other synthetics irritate the skin around the thighs, elbows, knees, wrists, ankles, or feet, especially if they are worn tightly. On the other hand, wool, silk, rubber, or leather may cause skin sensitization because of chemicals used as finishing agents, such as dyes, or chemicals to produce permanent creases, or to act as water repellents.

Treatment consists in eliminating the suspected item of clothing and replacing it with a nonallergic one. Patch tests done to detect the exact chemical nature of the allergen are not worth their expense.

The safest way to dress an atopic child is to have him wear undergarments and socks of pure cotton. Over these garments and socks he can wear any kind of material safely.

Summary of the Main Types of Eczema

Below are the differential diagnostic features of diaper rash, cradle cap, atopic eczema, and contact or hand eczema.

Diagnostic Features of the Main Types of Eczema

	Diaper rash	Atopic eczema	Cradle cap	Hand eczema
Age of onset	Very early	3 months	1–2 months	4–5 years
Family history of allergy	None	Frequent	None	None
Type of skin	Any	Dry	Oily	Any
Localization of lesion	Genital area	Flexures of arms and legs	Scalp and chest	Hands
Skin tests	Negative	Often positive	Negative	Negative
Patch tests	Negative	Negative	Negative	Positive

A Case History: Hand Eczema or Contact Dermatitis

Subject: L.B. (female)

Age: 12 years

Symptoms: Swollen, itchy, and blistered hands, present for many years.

History: L.B. suffered from eczema up to the age of three years. At nine years she developed poison ivy dermatitis at camp. Also, when washing dishes each night at home, the same symptoms appeared.

Diagnosis: Contact or "housewife" dermatitis.

Treatment: An allergist advised a change in detergents, but this was unsuccessful. A silicone cream applied to the hands did not improve her condition to any degree, either. Another allergist advised: (1) When washing dishes, to wear two pairs of gloves—a cotton glove under a rubber glove tied at the wrist with a rubber band; (2) while washing her hands to use Aveeno Bar or Lowilla Cake instead of regular soap; (3) to take antihistamines by mouth for the itch; (4) to apply cortisone cream to her hands at night.

    Three weeks later, L.B.'s hands had completely cleared up. The symptoms recurred only when L.B. used detergents without wearing gloves.

Soaps and Baths for the Eczematous Baby

Soap, a mixture of fatty acids with sodium salts, comes in either solid or liquid forms, and in different colors and odors, but all forms serve one purpose, that of cleaning a dirty skin. All soaps abrade the skin slightly. But while a normal skin can withstand that abrasion, the eczematous skin cannot. Washing an eczematous skin with ordinary soap and water removes a thin layer of fat that normally prevents the evaporation of water from the skin's inner layers and acts as a shield against outside irritants as well. The cleaning of this type of skin must be achieved without abrading it, and it needs, therefore, a special regime.

The ideal regime consists of *not* bathing the baby with any soap or water at all, but rather using Cetaphil lotion twice daily, applying it liberally and rubbing it in until it foams. It should then be wiped off gently with a soft cloth, leaving a film of the Cetaphil on the skin. If Cetaphil lotion is not available, then the child should be washed with Lowilla Cake or Aveeno Bar.

If Cetaphil lotion, Aveeno Bar, and Lowilla Cake are not available, then the child may have to use some special soaps, a different kind for different conditions. If the skin is extremely dry, the use of a superfatted soap, such as Basis or Dove, may serve to deposit some oil on it; if the skin is infected, a soap with an antibacterial agent, such as that in Dial, Safeguard, or Zest, may serve to reduce the amount of bacteria present on it. Antibacterial soaps, however, have their shortcomings. They sensitize the skin to light and make it prone to sunburn; also, if the antibacterial agent is an iodine preparation, the soap becomes doubly dangerous because iodine is a strong irritant to inflamed skin. Bubble baths with antibacterial agents are dangerous to girls, because they may cause urinary tract infection and vaginal irritation.

After the bath, no fatty lubricants should be allowed on the skin. Inflamed areas should be medicated with vioform-cortisone ointment, while undue infection should be controlled with erythromycin (an antibiotic), by mouth, and itching counterbalanced by Benadryl (an antihistamine), also by mouth. A baby's skin will remain clear on this regime for months. It is essential, however, that the baby never be bathed more than once weekly and that he continue to use only Cetaphil lotion, Aveeno Bar, or Lowilla Cake soaps for many years.

Parents must learn how to bathe an eczematous baby. The best time to do that is in the evening, when the baby has an empty stomach before the last meal of the day. Bathing the child at this hour will ensure a good night's sleep for both baby and parents because warm water relaxes the tension in the baby and enables him to fall asleep quickly. The baby has to have his bath in his own bedroom because it is dust free, contains his hypoallergenic soaps, his oils, and his clothing, and is ideally far from the kitchen and its odors.

The water of the bathtub must be around 90 to 95°F., and kept at that temperature with a bath thermometer. If the bottom of the tub is slippery, a diaper can be laid on it.

While the eczematous baby should not be bathed more than once weekly, the diaper area may be sponged more often. If the eczematous baby has cradle cap as well, his head and face are not to be bathed with water and soap at all, but simply cleaned with baby oil.

To sponge the baby, the parent should use a cotton washcloth dipped in clear warm water and nonallergenic soap. When the soaping is done, another washcloth should be used to wipe the soap off. The baby must then be dried—that is, blotted, never rubbed—with a soft bath towel. After drying the baby, the parent should clean his nostrils and ears with Q-Tips. If his skin is dry, he should be oiled; if it is oily, he should be powdered. The navel must look clean, and not red or infected.

The Effect of Sun Rays on the Skin of the Eczematous Baby

Sun rays contain an invisible ray, the ultraviolet ray, which penetrates the skin and causes inflammation with blisters, destruction of the skin, peeling, and formation of a dark pigment. This pigment indicates whether a child has gotten a healthy suntan or a sunburn. The amount of pigment formed from sunburn varies with the altitude of a location, the atmospheric pollution of the area, the color and thickness of the baby's skin, and the presence of water and snow in the vicinity. Areas located in high mountains have thin air, which cannot sufficiently shield a baby against ultraviolet rays; clouds and polluted air scatter these rays and make them weaker; dark, healthy, thick skin is less susceptible to being burned by these rays than white, thin skin; water and snow reflect ultraviolet rays just as a mirror does, and thus intensify their strength.

How to Sun an Eczematous Baby

Moderate exposure of a baby to the sun is healthy. To increase the tolerance of a light-skinned baby, one has to start with a two-minute exposure and increase by two minutes every day to a maximum of thirty minutes, dividing each day's quota between back and stomach positions. Reactions, which are stronger if the sunning is on a beach, because of reflected rays, will show up a few hours after sunning. While on the beach, the eczematous baby has to be protected not only from the sun, but from hot wind as well, because hot wind is as harsh on the skin as sun rays.

How to Avoid Sunburn

The most effective method of avoiding sunburn in an eczematous child is to apply on the skin a sunscreen that "blocks," "absorbs," or "scatters" some or all of the ultraviolet rays. Such screens are made basically of a chemical called PABA. This is incorporated in creams, ointments, or lotions sold commercially under such names as Pre-Sun and Pebanol. Complete protection from the sun's rays is accomplished by the application of an opaque substance, such as talcum powder or zinc oxide, which do not let any rays seep in at all. Such substances, however, should be reapplied after contact with water, because they may be washed away. The eyes are easy to protect from sun rays with dark glasses.

The disadvantages of "sun screens" are (1) that creams, lotions or powders may contain chemicals to which the eczematous child may be sensitive, and (2) that the ointment or the powder in which the screens are incorporated may clog the glands of the skin and aggravate the eczema.

Some camps in cold areas use sun lamps to promote general health. For use with eczematous children, these lamps should be mechanically timed to shut off at a reduced time span, since an eczematous skin can easily be burned in the exposure time regularly allowed for a child with normal skin.

Treatment of Sunburn

Burns come in three degrees: a first degree, in which the skin reddens only and will heal without leaving a scar; a second degree, in which it blisters; and a third degree, in which the damage goes beyond the skin. It takes several hours for even a first-degree burn to show, so a mother should rather underexpose her baby to the sun than watch for the skin to redden in order to tell whether her baby has been sunburned or not. A superficial burn can be taken care of by the parents: compresses of a saline solution can be used to soothe the pain of the burned area, and antiseptic-anesthetic skin lotions are healing. Blistering areas, however, need more attention, and should be handled by a doctor.

Prickly Heat and Its Prevention

Prickly heat is caused by perspiration resulting from high temperatures and excessive humidity. It shows up as a rash of tiny pink pimples and patches of pinkish skin confined to the neck and shoulder area. To avoid it, the baby should be dressed lightly, with loose clothing, in summer, and kept cool. If prickly heat does occur, the baby is to be bathed with cornstarch baths and powdered afterward. The powder should not be sprinkled directly from the container on the baby because the baby may inhale it. First, the powder must be shaken in the hand and then put on the baby, avoiding the eyes, nostrils, and hands; otherwise, the baby may rub the powder in his eyes.

HIVES

"Hives" or "urticaria" is the name given to itchy wheals that develop on the skin; "angioedema" is the name given to these wheals when they develop underneath the skin. The edema, or swelling, which gives the disease its name (angioedema) is caused by an allergic reaction in which histamine is released in the skin or underneath it. This release of histamine dilates the capillaries and allows some of their serum to ooze into the surrounding tissues to form wheals. These wheals itch intensely, and may either be limited to a small area of the body, such as the feet or the palms of the hands, or may join together and form big geographic figures called *giant hives*. Hives do not last more than forty-eight hours, and usually disappear without leaving a trace. Newly formed hives, however, may appear in other parts of the body.

Hives may be caused by an allergy to foods, drugs, infection, physical factors, or emotions.

Foods that frequently cause hives are chocolate, egg, fish, fresh fruit, nuts, shellfish, tomato, mustard, spices, and food additives. The drugs that cause hives are penicillin and aspirin. However, hormones, sulfa drugs, antibiotics, dyes, horse serum, iodides, laxatives, phenacetin, and tranquilizers may all cause hives, too.

The infections that cause hives are of a viral, bacterial, fungal, spirochetal, or parasitic (worms) nature. Such infections may reside in the tonsils, teeth, sinuses, ears, or gastrointestinal tract.

Physical factors that may cause hives are heat, cold, sun rays, or mechanical pressure. Hives caused by cold are especially dangerous; they may bring about a massive release of histamine in the body of a child who is swimming in cold water, and drowning may result. To avoid this, such children should be desensitized against cold. Pressure caused by tight straps, waistbands, girdles, and so forth may cause local hives. Sun rays cause solar hives, or hives brought about by the ultraviolet rays of the sun. Such hives appear on every exposed part of the body.

Rare causes of hives are (1) hives caused by a serum sickness brought about by an injection of immunized horse serum, which appears one week after the injection; or (2) hives caused by inhalants, such as dust, pollen, or molds. These respond to specific desensitization.

The diagnosis of hives in children does not require any skin testing. Children usually suffer from acute hives, which are normally caused by known allergies to a food (for example, shellfish) or a drug (penicillin).

The prevention of hives consists in avoiding their cause. The treatment of hives requires an adrenalin injection, and antihistamines by mouth.

Chronic Hives

When hives persist for a period of two months or more, they are called, arbitrarily, *chronic hives*. This is a symptom complex in which many factors join hands to perpetuate the disease. To uncover these factors we need an allergic history, a physical examination, a laboratory work-up, and a good follow-up.

The history and physical examination should be specific: (1) the presence of a dry skin; (2) atopic diseases (asthma, eczema, perennial rhinitis); (3) allergy to light, cold, heat, exertion, sweating; (4) allergy to metals used to repair dental cavities; (5) infections in the urinary tract or the feet (athlete's foot); (6) allergy to drugs (penicillin or aspirin); (7) emotional stability. The laboratory work-up should contain a urine examination, a stool examination for worms, a CBC, a sed rate, intracutaneous testing for inhalants, and a test for sensitivity to cold and heat. An elimination diet should take the place of testing for foods, because testing is unreliable.

It is very rare to find a child with chronic urticaria whose disease persists after an accurate study.

Summary of the Causes of Hives

1. Allergic factors

   Foods. Any food may cause hives, but the most common are:
   Milk and milk products (cheese, yogurt, etc.)
   Shellfish
   Fish
   Nuts
   Chocolate
   Tomatoes
   Eggs
   Peanuts and peanut products (butter)
   Strawberries
   Citrus fruits

   Drugs and chemicals. Any drug may cause hives, but the most common are penicillin and aspirin.

   Inhalants (pollen, fungi, animal dander)
   Contactants

2. Endogenous factors:
   Infections
   Parasites
   Endocrine disturbances

3. Physical factors:
   Cold
   Heat
   Sun
   Dermographism (writing on skin)

4. Miscellaneous rare organic factors

5. Emotional factors

6. Hereditary factors (hereditary angioedema)

SKIN DISORDERS AND EMOTIONS

Among all the skin disorders of atopic children, two acquire strong emotional overtones when they become chronic. These are eczema and hives.

Emotions in Chronic Eczema

Because the skin of an eczematous baby is more delicate and less horny than that of an adult, it may act as a mirror that can express the emotions of the body that lies underneath it. Fear, anger, shame, guilt, and excitement show up on the skin as pallor, sweating, or blushing. This comes about because both the baby's mind and his skin need each other to mature physically and emotionally. The fondling of the mother, the temperature changes, as well as the sensation of pain, stimulate the nerve endings of the skin and achieve a healthy inter-relationship between mind and skin.

Should the baby have an ugly discolored eczematous skin, the mother may stop her stroking of the skin, and thus hamper the emotional growth of the child. However, some eczematous children seem to need their long periods of skin scratching and stroking because this soothes their guilt feelings, allays their separation anxieties, and keeps them more infantile. Subconsciously, this is in compliance with the needs of their mothers, who may want their children to depend on them. Nevertheless, constant itching and scratching, even though done to resolve an emotional problem, creates a feeling of anger, frustration, and rebellion in a baby who finds himself caught in a turmoil from which he cannot escape.

Did the chicken lay the egg, or did the egg hatch into a chicken? Are confused emotions the result of the faulty upbringing of a child who has an abnormal skin? Or is the defective skin an expression of an emotionally disturbed mind? Maybe there is something of both in the eczematous child. A tranquilizer, such as Atarax or Vistaril, should form an integral part of the treatment of eczema in a child.

Emotions in Chronic Hives

Many children with chronic hives are brought to an allergist for treatment. They are either subsequently channeled to a psychiatrist or have the allergist serve as a therapist as well. The latter situation is in many ways optimum, as it takes advantage of the allergic study of the child and the already existing relationship between doctor and child.

Chronic hives is an allergic disease easily influenced by psychic stress. Exposure to allergens creates an allergic reaction, which causes the formation of chemicals that circulate in the blood, deposit themselves in the skin, and form hives which generate an urge to scratch when they reach a nerve ending. Psychogenic factors take over then, and set in motion a scratch-itch-scratch cycle. This causes a discomfort way out of proportion to any discomfort generated by the allergic reaction. It is presumed in such cases that feelings of anxiety and guilt manifest themselves in this form of self-punishment.

The psychic component that aggravates chronic hives responds to assurance, support, and the encouragement of self-esteem. Its treatment does not necessarily have to be done by a psychiatrist. Short-term psychotherapy could be supplied by the allergist, who may deal with the current issues and will not attempt major personality changes.

3 The Problems of the Atopic Baby During His Second Year

UPPER RESPIRATORY INFECTIONS AND ALLERGIES

Acute

A newborn baby has antibodies in his blood that protect him against respiratory infections. These antibodies, which he gets from his mother while he is still in the womb, are used up during the first year of life and leave him exposed to infections during the early part of his second year, until he makes enough antibodies of his own. During this interim period, the baby's respiratory infections become frequent and cause inflammations that erode his respiratory mucosa. These erosions permit the passage of minute particles of dead bacteria into his blood. These particles become allergens, which first sensitize the baby against the bacteria, and then create an allergy that manifests itself by frequent recurrences of colds and wheezing in the chest each time the baby is exposed to the same bacteria.

Allergy to bacteria is a controversial subject because testing for bacteria is not reliable and the diagnosis is clinical. Some criteria, however, give a clue to bacterial allergy:

1. The disease is frequent among atopic babies.

2. Babies with bacterial allergy suffer from other kinds of allergies besides the one to bacteria.

3. The disease improves with antibiotics.

4. The disease is worsened by injections of the bacteria that provoke it.

5. The disease improves with the removal of the usual sites of these bacteria (tonsils or adenoids).

Chronic

Acute upper respiratory infections disappear in two or three days unless there is a reason for them to last longer, or to recur. When they do last long or recur, they are called *chronic*. They may have become chronic because an allergy to a food or to an inhalant has sustained them. They are made worse by dry air, which comes about from overheating houses and apartments during winter. A house or an apartment that is heated to 68°F. or more needs a humidifier, because dryness acts like a sponge, absorbing the moisture of the mucosa of the nose, sinuses, and lungs. As this mucosa dries up, it becomes brittle and cracks, thus permitting the germs that lie above it to penetrate its interior and there multiply rapidly. To prevent this from happening, humidity has to be added to the air of the home. Boiling pans of water or putting receptacles filled with water above the radiator is not enough; the adequate humidification that is necessary can only be obtained by means of a humidifier of sufficient capacity, and with an accurate mechanism for automatic control. A medium-sized room requires about one gallon of water daily, and a three-room house ten to twenty gallons. If the house accumulates too much moisture because it is tightly sealed, an exhaust fan or an outside air intake may reduce moisture to desired levels. Houses that are not equipped with central humidification may need a portable electronic cold-air vaporizer for the bedroom, along with a hygrometer such as the Skuttle or the Taylor Humiguide to measure its humidity level. Cold air vaporizers, however, emit a fine white dust that is caused by the minerals dissolved in the water of the mist. This dust may accumulate in the air and on the furniture, and cause an irritative cough.

Humidification, air-conditioning, and heating problems in the house of an atopic child are extremely important issues that should not be handled by anyone who is not reputable and reliable.

Sinusitis

If an atopic baby gets more than seven "colds" during one year, he is getting more than his share of them. This may be due to a complication of the "cold" manifesting itself in the sinuses. Sinuses are cavities built around the nose and connected by small openings to its interior. They are not well developed at birth, but keep enlarging with the years to reach a maximum at puberty. Their lining, or mucosa, is covered with small filaments called *cilia*. These keep moving to create a flow of mucus from the sinuses to the nose.

The cilia of the nose then take over, and push the mucus to the esophagus, where it is eliminated. An increased quantity of "colds" increases the amount of mucus in the nose. This increased quantity of mucus cannot drain easily through the nose, so it pushes itself back into the sinuses, where it causes an inflammation.

The symptoms of sinusitis are some tenderness, swelling, and pain around the sinus area; a discharge with a foul odor from the nose; stuffiness; a diminished sense of smell; headaches; malaise; fever; and at times a toothache. These symptoms may follow an acute or chronic respiratory infection, a vasomotor disturbance caused by allergy, or an endocrine disturbance caused by hypothyroidism.

To diagnose a sinusitis, a doctor needs a thorough history with a physical examination; a transillumination—that is, the introduction of a small light bulb in the mouth of the child to illuminate his sinuses and observe if there are opacities there; an allergic work-up; and X rays of the sinuses.

The treatment of sinusitis consists of general supportive medications with tonics and vitamins, antibacterial therapy for the infections, and antiallergic measures. This treatment, however, must be accompanied by sinus drainage through steam inhalation, local heat, mechanical suction of the mucus from the sinuses, adequate fluid intake, vasoconstrictors taken by mouth or applied locally to the nose, and removal of chronically infected tonsils, polyps, or adenoids, which may be clogging the opening of the sinus into the nose and obstructing the natural flow of the mucus from the sinus to the nose.

The Nose Drip of the Allergic Child

An allergic child constantly secretes mucus from the lining of his nose and sinuses. As we have mentioned, this watery substance is pushed backwards to the esophagus by cilia attached to the cells of the lining. When the secretions become thick and abundant, for the reasons outlined below, instead of the constant flow of mucus we get thick drops of a sticky substance that the filaments find hard to push back. They remain in their place, and as they accumulate they begin to drop like small beads on the esophagus. This causes an irritative cough, which is a source of considerable nuisance.

The conditions that cause the mucus to become thick and abundant are:

1. Allergies to dust, pollen, molds, foods, and so forth, which increase the secretions of the lining of the nose and make them thicker.

2. Low-grade infections in the nose and sinuses, and allergy to the bacteria that cause such infections.

3. Nonspecific irritants of the lining of the nose and sinuses such as tobacco; excessive dryness of the air of the house due to overheating; overuse of nose drops that irritate the linings and push the secretions backwards; emotional disturbances that work on the sympathetic nervous system and cause an increase in nasal secretions; mechanical obstructions to the drainage of the sinuses through a deviated septum; endocrine deficiencies of a hypothyroid nature, which cause a dry and thick mucosa to secrete thick fluid.

Some ways to treat this condition:

1. Find out the allergic cause of the trouble through an accurate

history and testing, then eliminate it and desensitize against it if that is possible.

2. Give KI drops (saturated solution of potassium iodide) to soften the mucus and make it watery and therefore easy to expel. This medicine, which is better taken with milk to mask its acid taste, has to be changed every two weeks because during this time the iodine evaporates and the solution loses its potency. The dosage is ten drops in a tablespoonful of milk four times daily after meals for an adult. For children: one drop per year of age, three or four times daily. Some children cannot tolerate KI drops, and may develop either a rash or a swollen parotid gland. In that case, stop the medicine and contact the doctor for a substitute.

3. Let the child sleep with a high pillow, as opposed to a flat one, to get some symptomatic relief.

4. In winter, have a vaporizer going in the bedroom all night.

5. Use antibiotics on and off to control the frequent secondary infections in the sinuses that promote the drip.

6. The removal of polyps from the nose area, the mechanical suction of its mucus, and the application in the nose of packs containing vasoconstrictors, all facilitate sinus drainage and diminish the nose drip.

7. In general, oral medication and allergic desensitization give better results than local treatment in controlling a drip.

8. Give large doses of vitamin C. A lot has been written about the use of vitamin C in the prevention of colds. Although this is a necessary vitamin, and one that should be added to the diet of the atopic baby, we have no scientific proof that high doses of this vitamin prevents colds.

9. Last but not least, the parent has to bear in mind that the nose drip and the cough that comes with it are perfectly harmless and should, at their worst, be considered only a nuisance. If the condition is too nerve-racking for the parent, he or she can use tranquilizers.

But even though a postnasal discharge in itself is not harmful, and usually has little significance, it must not always be dismissed lightly, as it may be a sign of a more serious disease. Chronic bronchitis, laryngitis, nervous tics, tumors of the lung, enlarged mediastinal nodes, bronchiectasis, and emphysema must all come into consideration in the differential diagnosis.

Allergy or Infection?

Sometime around the second year of an atopic baby's life the question arises as to whether the allergies of the child are precipitating his infections or whether his infections are promoting his allergies by opening the door to them through an eroded and inflamed respiratory mucosa. A parent must be able to resolve this dilemma all alone.

A child who has no family history of allergy, no history of feeding difficulties, no atopic dermatitis, no undue nose clogging, no croup, no nosebleeds, and no chestiness is a child who suffers from infection. A child who has a family history of allergy, has suffered from feeding problems (colic, vomiting, diarrhea, canker sores), skin problems (dry skin, bad diaper rashes, eczema, contact dermatitis), upper respiratory problems (swollen nasal mucosas, congested eyes, itchy nose, breathing through the mouth, wheezing), who is worse during certain particular seasons (winter for dust-sensitive children, summer for pollen-sensitive children), is an allergic child who is developing secondary infections. However, the differential diagnosis is not always easy, because the relationship of allergy to infection may become very intimate. Dr. A. Horesh cites these sayings on the subject:

Recurrent upper respiratory infection is one of the most important, least understood and consequently most neglected of the allergic diseases of infancy and childhood.[1] Respiratory infection and respiratory allergy walk hand in hand.[2] That allergy increases susceptibility to infection is axiomatic.[3] Allergy to milk and dairy

1. Jerome Glaser.
2. James Hill.
3. Frederic Speer.

products should be suspected when a child has repeated upper respiratory tract infections.[4] The history of repeated respiratory or middle ear infections may provide the first clue to the diagnosis of allergic disease, particularly in small children.[5]

4. Gerrard.
5. Bellanti.

4 The Problems of the Atopic Baby During His Third Year

INHALANT ALLERGY IN THE BEDROOM

A baby's room contains articles that naturally appertain to it, such as clothing, cosmetics worn by the mother, mattress fillings, carpeting, and so forth. These articles break down and fly into the air as minute light pieces called *inhalants*. Following is a list of bedroom inhalants that may evoke an allergic reaction as a child breathes them: orrisroot, kapok, cottonseed, flaxseed, tobacco, pyrethrum, and house dust.

Orrisroot

Orrisroot is a powder obtained from the root of the iris flower, and is used as a basis for many kinds of cosmetics. It is usually brought into the bedroom by the parent in the form of cosmetics or other drugstore items.

These cosmetics or drugstore items contain orrisroot:

Face powder	Sunburn lotion	Scented soap
Shaving cream	Sachet	Bath salts
Facial cream	Rouge	Hair tonic
Toothpaste or powder	Perfume	Shampoo
	Lipstick	

As far as cosmetics are concerned, a mother should discard her old powder puff and use "nonallergenic" cosmetics that contain no orrisroot. Many cosmetics manufacturers have become aware of the dangers of allergy to orrisroot, and are no longer including it in their products. Among these are Elizabeth Arden, Armand's Symphony, Almay, Max Factor (Pancake), Marcelle, Botay, and Mary Dunhill. And it is best to use the nonscented items in these cosmetics lines.

House Dust

By far the most important inhalant yet to be discussed is house dust. House dust is not the dust blown in from the street, but rather a complex substance produced by the action of mites that feed on the scales shed by the human skin over mattresses, carpeting, and clothing in old, damp bedrooms. It may contain traces of mildew, animal dander, a wide variety of lint, insect waste, tobacco, and so forth. Its makeup can vary widely, depending on the family's living habits, house construction, geographic location, climate, and many other unforeseen factors. Babies are easily sensitized to this complex substance, and they should avoid it at all costs. Special procedures in building a model house for the allergic child and also in keeping his bedroom clean and free of dust must be followed. The procedures, which are extensive, are detailed on pages 66–70.

A Case History: Allergy to Dust
Subject: R.B.

Age: 3 years

Habitat: 5-story Bronx tenement

Symptoms: Clogged nose for a period of one year; mouth breathing; slight deafness in both ears; frequent upper respiratory infections.

Diagnosis: A skin test for dust was strongly positive. R.B.'s pediatrician prescribed nose drops, antihistamines, and desensitization against dust for a period of six months.

Comments: Response to treatment was poor. As a result, R.B.'s mother consulted an allergist, who suggested the following:

1. R.B. must move from his old house and stay with an aunt living in a new home in a nearby area. Old houses contain more dust than new ones.

2. Antihistamines and nose drops were to be discontinued, and saline drops to be instilled in the nose instead. (The antihistamines dried up the nose secretions and excessive nose drops irritated the nasal mucosa.)

3. An electrostatic air purifier and humidifier was to be installed in R.B.'s bedroom to make it free of dust, animal hair, and odors, and also to provide enough moisture in its air.

4. The injections of dust were to be started again, but in weaker doses.

One year later, the polyps had cleared from R.B.'s nose; he no longer found it necessary to breathe through his mouth; his respiratory infections had decreased. The dust injections were continued for another year to prevent a recurrence.

Kapok

This is a tree whose fibers are used as mattress filling and in life preservers because they are moisture resistant. Kapok is being used less frequently now since the discovery of foam rubber and other synthetics.

Cottonseed

These are the seeds that remain attached to the small cotton fibers. They are used in padding cushions, sofas, and quilts, and when pressed they produce an oil that is used in cooking and in packing sardines. When ground their flour is incorporated in fertilizers or animal feed; milk from cows fed with cottonseed is dangerous to the atopic child if he is sensitive to it.

Flaxseed

Flax, a plant of the genus *Linum* is widely grown for the

production of linseed oil and linen fiber. It may cause allergies when eaten, inhaled, or by direct contact. Foods that contain flaxseed are flaxseed tea and the milk of cows fed flaxseed. Inhalants that contain flaxseed are wave sets, shampoos, hair tonics, furniture polish, linseed oil, linoleum, soft soap, printer's ink, and some depilatories. Clothes made of flax or linen are linen handkerchiefs, damask, sheeting, cambric, and toweling.

Tobacco

Smoking is irritating to the lungs because it neutralizes their natural defenses by paralyzing their cilia. These tiny hairlike structures that line the respiratory mucosa trap dirt and bacteria so they can be pushed away from the lungs toward the esophagus. Smoking also hampers the work of the macrophages, which are the "vacuum-cleaner" cells of the lungs and stops them from disposing of harmful substances. This is followed by destruction of the lung tissue and pre-emphysema. Furthermore, smoking may cause allergy to the tobacco leaf and to the many ingredients mixed with it.

Pyrethrum

Pyrethrum is the principal ingredient of some insecticides. It is related to ragweed, and those children who are allergic to ragweed should avoid it. Kilit, sold by the National Allergic Sales Company of New York City, is an insecticide free of pyrethrum.

Miscellaneous Inhalants

Certain items are a potential source of trouble if they are accidentally found in the child's bedroom. Examples are glue, vegetable gums present in wave sets, hand lotion, candies, toothpaste, naphthalene, gasoline, kerosene, perfume, foods, or freshly cut flowers.

A MODEL HOME FOR THE ALLERGIC CHILD

When the parents of an allergic child have the opportunity to build a new home, careful planning can greatly reduce its potential as a collector of allergens. These suggestions will help to build in advantages seldom found in a "ready built" house.

1. Don't put the garage under the house unless absolutely necessary; certainly not on the same side as the allergic child's bedroom.

2. A workshop would be less offensive in the garage than in the cellar, where sawdust, paint fumes, and so forth can rise through the house.

3. Install a well-filtered and humidified central air-conditioning system.

4. A central vacuum system will greatly reduce the risk of recirculating dust. Its motor and collection tank should be located in a sealed furnace room.

5. Don't skimp on the kitchen exhaust fan, as this must quickly remove all cooking smoke and vaporized oils before they permeate the house.

6. The oil or gas furnace should be in a sealed room accessible only from the outside to avoid the circulation of fumes.

7. The clothes dryer should be in an enclosed room and vented to the outside.

8. Plan to have no closets inside the allergic child's bedroom. They are gathering places for dust and allergens brought in by the clothes.

9. Make sure that the child is not allergic to the insulation materials selected.

10. Hot water or electric heat serve best because they won't dry out the house or blow dust around.

11. For floors, sheet vinyl is better than vinyl squares. A floor of squares has many feet of joining seams which may collect dust and dirt. Cement floors should be treated with a paint to waterproof them and prevent the shedding of cement dust.

12. Sheet vinyl is best for bathroom walls. Small grouted tiles are hard to clean and will grow mold.

13. Avoid recreation areas below ground level, as they are breeders of mold. (No cellar is best of all.)

The Allergic Child's Model Bedroom

The kind of bedroom that the allergy-prone child should have is of the utmost importance in preventing allergy to house dust. The child's room must be weatherstripped, with all wall and floor cracks sealed. There should be an air-filtering device or an electronic precipitator installed in it. Big devices that can remove the dust as well as control the humidity of the whole house work better than window devices, which can only perform a limited service. These larger devices are becoming less costly each year, and they are fully tax deductible if installed with a doctor's prescription. Electronic room units are manufactured by such companies as West Bend, Sunbeam, McGraw-Edison, and Montgomery Ward, while General Electric, Westinghouse, Emerson Electric, Trion, Luxaire, Fedders, and Chrysler Air-Temp are among some of the reputable brands of central system air cleaners.

The mechanical removal of dust from the room should be done daily with a damp cloth or an oil mop, and later the room must be aired. It should also be left closed when it is not being used. Needless to say, the child must be brought to another room during the cleaning process.

The type of heating used for the bedroom is very important. An electric heater is preferable to hot-air heating, but if the latter is already installed, its outlets should be covered with cheesecloth or gauze.

The furniture in the room must be very simple, to make its scrubbing and cleaning easier. There need be only a chair for an adult to sit on, and a high table that has a few drawers for safety pins, the child's vitamin drops, and some nonallergenic soaps. (Other necessary items for the bedroom are found in the medicine cabinet. These are a rectal thermometer, Tylenol drops [instead of baby aspirin, because this is less allergenic], petroleum jelly, a hot-water bottle, a rubber ear syringe, plastic-packed cotton balls, a bath thermometer, one forceps, adhesive tape, Band-aids, a bottle warmer, baby lotion, baby powder, zinc ointment and baby scales. None of these items is a major source of house dust, and they can be kept safely in the child's medicine cabinet or the bedroom.) A washable plastic pail with a cover for discarded diapers is also needed near the table.

The child's crib or bed must be simple, with no pillows or comforters, and must contain a mattress filled with foam rubber. If the mattress does not contain foam rubber, it must be enclosed in a zippered plastic cover, which can be bought ready made in an allergy-free store or made to order to fit the existing mattress. Ready-made encasings and mattresses such as Protecto Dust Encasings and Modern Foam Mattress can be purchased from Allergy Free Products for the Home, P.O. Box 345, 1162 West Lynn Street, Springfield, Mo. 65801. The sheets of the crib or bed must be of a washable cotton fabric and the blankets of Orlon, Dacron, or Acrilan. Washable, lintless rag rugs made of nylon or other synthetics may be used on the floor of the room. There should be no upholstery or pads made from animal hairs under the carpet, and the carpet must not contain any wool. Cotton curtains, as well as roll-up window shades, are better than drapes for the windows. Toys are allowed in the room provided they are made of iron, wood, or plastic, and have no stuffing inside. They are to be scrubbed and cleaned together with the rest of the furniture.

The child's room must be pleasant. If the child dislikes his room and considers his confinement there as a disciplinary measure designed to limit his freedom, the emotional trauma that may result may be worse than the physical protection he gets. The room has to be decorated with gay colors in unusual designs, using ingenuity and imagination. It should also contain all that the child needs, since it is better to concentrate all effort and expense on one single room. It may have to be divided into two sections: one a sort of living room, where the child can do his homework, when he reaches school age, and watch TV, and the other for sleeping purposes. As an extra precautionary measure, the child must be made to wear a dust mask in his room for a day or two following any extensive painting or cleaning in it. A dust mask, which is the same as a hay fever mask, comes in lightweight disposable paper made by 3M Company, Dept. FH, P.O. Box 33686, St. Paul, Minn. 55101, or as a polyethylene painter's mask, which can be procured from the Allergist's Supply Company, 90-94 161 Street, Jamaica, N.Y. 11432.

Hazards of an Atopic Child's House

Remember, an atopic child is a child above all. Even though his own bedroom is allergy free, it—and his whole house—may still be a potential source of certain hazards. We mention them here even though they belong to pediatrics because they form part of the atopic child's life.

Small children who crawl explore their environment and put into their mouths anything they find along their way. Such material may consist of after-shave lotions, drugs, cleaning agents, cosmetics, dyes, glue, mothballs, matches, nail polish, rat poison, rubbing alcohol, vitamins, and wax. All these items are poisonous, as well as sensitizing.

For older children, parents must try to keep workshop and garage items out of easy reach, use lead-free paints in the house, teach the children to recognize the poison insignia of skull and crossbones, and check the yard for plants that have poisonous leaves or berries.

If the child is seen swallowing a poisonous item, or if its container is discovered empty, these symptoms may be expected: stains and burns around the mouth of the child, drowsiness, rapid breathing, vomiting, stomach pains, convulsions, and unconsciousness.

In such a situation, the first thing to do is to examine the label of the package, then call the nearest poison center in the area and take the child to the nearest hospital. For emergency situations, vomiting can be induced. The child must be given a teaspoonful of syrup of ipecac, and later a teaspoonful of activated charcoal as an antidote to the poison. Both of these items can be purchased without a prescription at any drugstore.

To prevent recurrence of such an accident, all medicines must be stored and locked in the medicine cabinet, all unused products discarded and all torn labels replaced.

The following phone numbers must be hung up by the telephone: physician, poison control center, hospital, first-aid squad, ambulance, druggist, police department, fire department, and neighbor.

5 The Problems
of the Atopic Child
During His Fourth Year

At four to five years of age most children are not yet in school on a full-time basis. The child spends his free time in his room, outside his apartment, or in the back yard of his house. The back yard area can be a tremendous source of allergy, especially if the child happens to live in the country. We reserve this chapter for a discussion of the animals found in the back yard, the shrubs that grow in it, and the insects that are likely to be found there.

ANIMALS

Epidermoids are the scales normally shed by animals with furs or feathers, and are highly sensitizing agents. Even though parents have been instructed not to bring any furry or feathered animals into the house, they might not be able to stop their child's contact with them in the homes of neighbors or in the back yard.

In one way or another, he may come across these animals: horses, chickens, dogs, cats, rabbits, sheep, goats, cows, rats, mice, monkeys, parrots, canaries, pigeons, and guinea pigs. Feeding rabbits, dogs, cats, and squirrels is a frequent pastime for many children, and so is playing with bird's nests. These habits should be discouraged, because animal hair and feathers are extremely potent creators of allergy, an allergy for which desensitization is not effective and avoidance is imperative.

Allergex is a preparation made to spray on pets to reduce the amount of scales and hair that the animal sheds. The author doubts that it can do this effectively, and prescribes it only on rare occasions, for psychological reasons—to quiet a house in the turmoil caused by the discovery that a very dear pet is the cause of allergy. Allergex is available from Allergy Free Products for the Home, P.O. Box 345, 1162 West Lynn Street, Springfield, Mo. 65801.

Birds

The feathers of live birds (chickens, ducks, geese, parrots, canaries, turkeys, and so forth), or the feathers used in stuffing pillows or quilts, are potent sensitizers that should be avoided regardless of the results of skin tests.

Besides acting as an allergen, feathers may harbor dust and molds. When in pillows, their proximity to the nose for eight hours each night makes them especially dangerous inhalants. It is imperative that an atopic child sleep on a nonallergenic pillow (foam, Dacron) whether in his home or away.

A parrot or a canary to which a child is emotionally attached may be allowed to remain in the house provided it is never introduced into the child's bedroom.

Horses

These are highly sensitizing animals that can quickly and frequently cause asthma and rhinitis. Smelling horse hair in a stable, or touching the clothes of a rider, or even walking at a distance from a horse, may give sensitivity reactions.

Sensitivity to horse serum usually goes along with sensitivity to horse hair. A child should not be given immunized horse serum if he is know to be sensitive to horse hair. He should be tested for horse serum, and if he gives a positive reaction, should be given immunized human serum instead. However, serum sickness is rare now because all children are being routinely immunized against tetanus, which previously required treatment with tetanus-immune horse serum.

Dogs

These are pets to which a child may become easily attached. Dogs have no sweat glands, and in the summer months their saliva runs out of their mouths over everything, including furniture. This saliva, together with their hair and skin scales, is highly sensitizing material that the atopic child should avoid.

A child who does not have a dog should not get one. If he has a dog and is attached to it, he should be allowed to keep it, but should not replace it when it dies. Until then, the dog should not enter the bedroom of the child, and should be kept out of the house as much as possible.

There are no safe breeds of dog. A child may be sensitive to a poodle but not to a collie, but this is no reason to change one kind of dog for another. Sensitivity catches up with the child, and he will be just as sick with the new dog. Although this may be heartbreaking for dog lovers, we have no better answer to the problem at the present time: an atopic child must try to live without a dog.

Cats

Cat hair is an extremely dangerous sensitizer, which can bring on coryza and asthma. It can be inhaled by a child even at a distance, and remains in a house for many days after the cat has left it.

Cat hair has a limited industrial use in the making of robes, coats, gloves, or toy animals. However, when such hair is properly sterilized, it loses its allergenic powers.

The leopard, panther, wildcat, jaguar, tiger, lion, and lynx belong to the cat family, and should, during a visit to the zoo, be avoided by the child who is sensitive to cats.

Rabbits

Children who have rabbits as pets may develop allergies on contact with them. On the other hand, rabbit hair used in bedding, upholstery, or clothing may cause eczema and coryza only when it is not properly dyed and sterilized before use.

Goats

The same warnings for rabbit hair also apply to goat hair. Mohair, alpaca, angora, and cashmere are names for goat hair used to make coats or sweaters.

Sheep

Wool is an important element in clothing. While refined and dyed woolen clothing does not cause allergies, coarse wool used for knitting, or wool in the process of being spun, may cause rhinitis, asthma, or eczema.

Rats and Mice

The hair of these rodents may cause allergies in children living in slum areas.

It has to be stressed to the parents of children who are sensitive to any of the above-mentioned animals again and again that the offender may not be a live animal. It may consist of an improperly processed fur, a mounted head of a buck, a tiger-hide throw, or a stuffed eagle.

What to Do When "The Pet Must Go"

When a child proves to be allergic to animal fur, feathers, dander, or saliva, our recommendation may have to be: "The pet must go."

It is a good idea to make certain that the departure of the pet is absolutely necessary. A trial can be made by boarding the pet elsewhere for two or three months and cleaning the house thoroughly. During this period, an allergic work-up may determine whether the pet is indeed the cause of the allergy. All breeds of cats and dogs are harmful, short hair as well as long hair. Nonallergenic breeds of dogs or cats do not exist.

With a child, there is bound to be an emotional wrench in the separation. A pet fulfills a need in that child's life, and to whisk it away summarily, without thoughtful staging or "replacement therapy," could have unfortunate consequences. If the pet is a dog, it may be a type that can be kept out of doors; the child might enjoy helping to build a dog house. However, the dog *must* remain outdoors, and under no circumstances should it be allowed to travel in a car or any other conveyance with the child.

If the family must part with a pet altogether, this can sometimes be done in stages:

1. Boarding the animal elsewhere, as during the work-up period, provides a break in the relationship that allows the child to be "weaned" away before the separation is made permanent.

2. It may be better to take the child away from the pet rather than the pet away from the child. Perhaps the child could be taken on a trip or be sent to camp or to stay with a relative while another home is found for the pet.

3. It is important that the child believe the pet will be happy. A picture of his new home or of other animals he will be with may help.

"Replacement therapy" can be all important. The initial shock to a child can be softened with an inanimate object, something to fill the gap while the child forgets. A new bike, a radio or phonograph may do it; most children will respond to the substitute in a relatively short time. (Do *not* substitute a stuffed pet for a live one, because this may cause allergic reactions.) And although fish do not provide the opportunity for love and affection that a dog or a cat does, a small aquarium may divert the child's attention during the initial departure period. Be certain the fish food or filtering elements do not introduce new allergens. Or if the child is one who shows unusual love for all animals and is affected considerably by the loss, transference may be brought about if the parents take an interest in, say, wild birds. Bird feeders and bird houses can be built. Bird watching or bird walks can be initiated, and books about birds can be bought. The child's room can be decorated with bird pictures.

Finally, the child may need a new "friend" most of all. Schoolmates should be invited home often.

Note: Desensitization against animal dander may be carried out against dogs, cats, or horses if some *exceptional circumstances* warrant it. These are (1) if the livelihood of the child's parents depends on handling animals (veterinarians or laboratory workers); (2) if the allergic symptoms are very mild, and the psychological trauma resulting from the removal of the animal is great; (3) where even casual contact with an animal leads to asthma.

ALLERGY TO BEES AND OTHER INSECTS

Bees are frequently found among trees and shrubs; they may cause serious allergic reactions when they bite or sting an atopic child. Other insects to be avoided are fleas, ants, spiders, mosquitoes, scorpions, wasps, hornets, and yellowjackets. Among the bees, only the honey bee will leave its stinger and venom sac in the skin of the child when it stings him. This is important, as the stinger and sac have to be removed before we start treating him for allergic reactions.

When stung by a bee or an insect, a child may have a normal reaction to that sting, characterized by pain, itching, and swelling in the area. This is to be treated with ice packs, a local application of calamine lotion, and antihistamines by mouth.

On the other hand, he may have a serious generalized reaction occurring fifteen to thirty minutes after the sting, which may be toxic or allergic in its nature or both. A toxic reaction may occur in a child who is not allergic to insect or bee venom, provided he has had many stings of the venom at the same time. Toxic symptoms include diarrhea, vomiting, fainting, unconsciousness, and even death. Allergic symptoms result from small quantities of venom. These include local reactions, as mentioned above, and systemic reactions, which are immediate or delayed and can be divided into three categories according to their intensity. Mild reactions are local hives, malaise, and anxiety. Moderate reactions are generalized hives, wheezing, nausea, and dizziness. Severe reactions are laryngeal edema, difficulty in breathing, marked weakness, disorientation, incontinence, cyanosis, shock, and death. Some allergic reactions may choose to manifest themselves in unorthodox ways, such as pains in the joints, temperature elevation, or internal bleeding.

The treatment of generalized reactions depends on their type, their time of onset, and their severity. The most dangerous allergic reaction is anaphylactic shock, and this has to be treated firmly and quickly. If this happens and the stinger is present, flick it off without squeezing the area. A tourniquet should then be tied above the place of the bite, and an injection of ⅓ cc. of adrenalin should be given in the site of the bite. If the child becomes cyanotic and has difficulty breathing, he should be given oxygen. If he does not respond to these two measures, he should be given another injection of adrenalin as well as a corticosteroid, and then he should be rushed to the nearest hospital.

A child who has had a severe local reaction to a venom is likely to have a more severe reaction in his next exposure to the same venom. He must therefore always carry his own drugs for emergencies. Furthermore, if his reaction was life threatening, he must have hyposensitization treatment for many years, not by a general practitioner, but by a Board-certified allergist. Such a child must wear a tag indicating he is allergic to insect or bee stings. Such tags can be ordered as a bracelet or metal medallion from the Medic Alert Foundation (P.O. Box 1009, Turlock, Calif. 95380). On these are engraved the medical problem of the wearer, his file number, the telephone number of Medic Alert's Central File, the address of the personal physician of the patient and his phone number, his nearest relatives, and so forth. All information can be gotten via a collect telephone call (twenty-four hours daily) to the Central File of the foundation (209 632-2371).

Protection Against Bees and Other Insects

The house of the child can be protected against bees and other insects by means of screens. In the back yard, bee hives are usually built in shrubs, in the ground, or high in trees. They should be destroyed by a professional exterminator who will hose or knock them down with a stick, and then spray the area with insecticide. The exterminator must keep visiting the back yard once a week to look for new hives, and also to see to it that the area is clean and free of open garbage cans and rotting foods, because these attract bees and insects.

The child must not wear clothes with flowery designs or walk barefoot, as these practices attract bees. He must be fed large amounts of vitamin B_1 (thiamine hydrochloride) during the summer months, because this vitamin gives a special odor to the body that bees hate and avoid. Furthermore, if he is allergic to bees, he must be skin tested and desensitized. The results of such treatment are not always gratifying, however.

Emergency Treatment by the Child Himself

As a last resort, if a doctor is not around, the allergic child should take care of himself when stung by a bee or an insect. He should always carry an emergency kit that contains tweezers to remove the venom sac, antihistamines, Isuprel tablets, and an adrenalin injection. He should start by removing the venom sac, then swallow the antihistamine tablet, and put the Isuprel tablet under his tongue. He should then call a parent who has been trained in giving injections or a nurse to give him his ready-to-use injection of adrenalin.

A Case History: Reaction to Bee Stings

Subject: C.L.

Age: 4 years

Personal History: C.L. is an atopic boy previously stung by bees on many occasions, but experiencing only local reaction, which increased in intensity each time.

Symptoms: Stung by a honey bee. Three or four minutes after the sting, C.L., who had been dressed in a bright, rough fabric, developed hives, difficulty in breathing, and cyanosis.

Treatment: C.L. was rushed to the nearest hospital where he was injected with .5 cc. of adrenalin and 1 cc. of Solu-Cortef (a cortisone preparation); he was also given oxygen by inhalation. He improved quickly, and was sent home after two hours.

Comments: The treatment was correct, and probably saved the child's life. C.L. had shown increasing local reactions to stings that led to a general catastrophic reaction. He should have been wearing a tag telling about his allergy to bee stings, and how this should be treated in an emergency.

He should have been given these instructions about avoiding bees and insects, even though it is hard to conceive that a four-year-old child can follow them:

1. If a bee approaches, he should not make a jerky or unexpected movement.

2. He should stay away from blossoming trees, trees with fermenting fruits, areas with drinking faucets, leftover food, or open garbage pails.

3. In summer, while in open spaces, he should wear simple, long-sleeved clothing with no floral designs. He should use no hair preparations or perfumes and avoid perspiration and fatigue. He

should always carry with him an insect-repelling bomb, and never play in a back yard that contains bee hives.

If the child is unable to follow the instructions, he should not play in the back yard till he reaches the more mature age of six or seven years.

POISON IVY

The poison ivy plant is a vine that climbs on nearby trees or walls and that can grow as a ground creeper or bush. Its leaf is composed of three leaflets, two of which are directly opposite each other. The leaflets are about three inches long, and their edges are either smooth or notched. The leaves are glossy green in summer and bear clusters of white flowers, which turn red in the fall and then become berries. The berries, which are about as large as raisins, are not poisonous to eat. The peak of incidence of ivy poisoning is in spring and summer, when outdoor activities are greatest, but contact with the plant may cause the disease even in winter. The poison ivy vine, its flowers, and its berries are all coated with a thin layer of a very potent oil that may cause a skin irritation. This irritation appears as an itchy red patch on the skin, which turns into a blister two to three hours after contact with the plant. The skin blisters may open up and "dribble" over adjacent parts of the body. This dribbling, however, does not cause new lesions. The whole area takes about two to three weeks to heal.

Two other plants, poison sumac and poison oak, are small shrubs that do not normally grow in back yards but may be found in fields. Because they are coated with the same oil that coats the poison ivy plant, they cause the same type of skin lesion as that of poison ivy. If poison ivy, poison sumac, or poison oak plants are burned, their oil evaporates. It may then cause irritation to the eye or nose of a sensitive child who may be many yards away. Furthermore, the same oil may stick to the hair of cats or other animals that roam in the back yard, and these may carry it inside the home of the child. Such indirect contamination remains dangerous for many months.

Prevention

To prevent contact with poison ivy, the plant must be completely eliminated from the back yard by using a commercial brush killer, which can be bought at hardware, drug, or farm supply stores. To kill the vine, apply the chemical thoroughly with a paint brush to the lower part of the plant only; there is no need to apply the paint to the upper part of the vine. The brush killer is best used in the fall or early spring, or when the plant is not actually growing. One application, if done correctly, kills the vine. Also, washing or dry cleaning the intermediaries that have come in contact with the plant —such as pets, shoes, clothing, tools, and so forth—is important, and so is the use of barrier creams (such as silicone) on the exposed areas of the body of the child when he is outdoors.

There is no way to prevent poison ivy allergy through desensitization. Desensitization against poison ivy, whether done by mouth or by injection, is a controversial issue, and we have no proof that it works. Some natural protection against poison ivy is acquired with age, and also with exposure. Older children get it less than younger children, and farmers and foresters are less sensitive to it than city dwellers. It is best avoided by staying away from it. If that is not possible, the exposed areas of the body have to be coated with a lather of yellow laundry soap that can be washed off later. Very few people are immune to poison ivy, and under proper conditions almost *everyone* can get the disease.

Treatment

After having touched poison ivy, a child should be washed with soap and water immediately. If blistering has already occurred, the affected area should be treated with soaks of normal saline. If the blisters have become infected, then 1:100 Burow's solution in tap water would serve better than saline. The soaking should be done with a white cloth dipped in the solution, then wrung out tightly and used on the affected area for half an hour each time, six times daily. A fresh solution of saline or Burow's solution should be used for each application. An antihistamine, such as Temaril syrup, should be given by mouth to calm the itching. If the lesions are extremely painful and extensive, corticosteroids may be given by mouth, although corticosteroids should always be used with extreme care.

6 The Problems of the Atopic Child During His Fifth and Sixth Years

SCHOOL

Going to school for the first time is an exciting experience for any child, and the parents, the school nurse, and the doctor must all cooperate and try to make this experience an especially pleasant one for the atopic child. A school should be a place free of worry and allergies, where a potentially sick child can develop his personality and increase his knowledge. Education should be the most important objective in going to school, and allergies should not stand in its way. Education for the atopic child should mean, above all, self-discipline, because he more than all the other children must accept his shortcomings, avoid sickness, and yet function well enough to achieve an educational level normal for his age.

Clothing

In winter, the atopic child who goes to school must be properly dressed, not with coarse woolen clothes, but with soft, dyed woolens or synthetics, all of which must be taken out of storage a few days before school and left in the fresh air outside the house. In this manner, any smell of mothproofing will disappear. Pockets should also be emptied and searched for moth balls.

Transportation

On cold winter days, the child must wear a mask so that he does not have to breathe cold air. These masks are manufactured by Carman Commodities, and are available in stores that sell allergy-free products. The mask should be worn in the street as well as in the school bus, to avoid exhaust fumes. In the bus, the child should try to sit near the driver, where the fumes are less prevalent. In case the bus has to follow a long and polluted city route to collect children, it may be safer to drive the child to school in a private, closed, and heated car. If that is being done, certain precautions must be taken. The child should enter the car before it has been started in order to avoid exposure to exhaust fumes. The fumes that come out of the car have to be controlled by steam-cleansing the engine yearly; checking the radiator, brake fluid, and gas caps for correct sealing; changing the crankcase valve frequently; adjusting the carburetor and automatic choke properly; inspecting the exhaust system for leaks; and not overfilling the gas tank. The seat covers of the car must be tightly sealed to help keep dust and molds from gathering inside the upholstery. Feather or kapok pillows should not be allowed in the car, nor any animal with fur or feathers. The car should be air conditioned, its windows should in any case be closed at all times, and the air vents found under the dashboard sealed with cheesecloth. The car should be vacuum cleaned often, and its interior surface and floor mats washed frequently. The windshield should be tinted. If this is impossible, the child should wear dark glasses to relieve his light-sensitive eyes. Smoking should never be allowed in the car.

While driving the child to school, the parents should keep the car route clean by bypassing the immediate vicinity of farms, refineries, industrial plants, or freshly tarred highways. Rush-hour traffic should be avoided, and a distance of four car lengths behind other vehicles should be kept in order to avoid inhalation of exhaust fumes. The following of diesel buses or trucks should be avoided, since they spew out chemical pollutants. The child should avoid riding in the car before 11:00 A.M. and after 6:00 P.M., as these are the periods of highest pollen concentration. Also, riding whenever the wind is blowing should be avoided to eliminate exposure to molds. When the car is being refilled with gas, the child should sit in it with the windows, of course, closed.

School Meals

An atopic child's meals should be prepared at home and taken to school in order to avoid the specific foods to which he may be allergic. In any case, shellfish and fish, peanut butter, fresh fruits, chocolate, and nuts should never be included in a child's lunch, as these foods are all highly allergenic. A list of the foods to which the child is allergic should be carried in his pocket at all times and a copy of it should be kept in the school cafeteria.

Activities

While in school, the allergic child should try to participate in normal physical activities. If normal activities lead him into trouble, he should avoid dusty playgrounds and heavy gym activities, as well as swimming in chlorinated pools. If he is an asthmatic, and prolonged exercise causes slight bronchospasm, an oral bronchodilator should be taken one hour before the exercise. If this is not enough, and prolonged exercise invariably causes strong asthma attacks, these exercise activities must be restricted to such exercises which require frequent intervals of rest, such as baseball, or the 100-yard dash. If this also causes asthma, then the child should take up only very light physical activities, such as building models, or playing table top games.

Colds

The teacher and the nurse should see to it that the child is never seated near someone who has a common cold. If by chance the child is surrounded by children with colds because of an epidemic, he must be made to wear a mask, provided this does not make him feel like an outcast.

Classes

The child should not erase blackboards or do cleaning chores that stir up dust, and should be seated in the back of the class. That way he does not have to inhale chalk dust and does not have to be near the flowers, pets, or plants that are usually situated in the front of the class.

The atopic child who is allergic to animals should try to avoid special class trips to museums, farms, zoos, racetracks, and parks, but if such trips are undertaken, special medication must be provided specifically for the trip. Although he should be made to socialize with his schoolmates, he should be careful in visits to them to avoid potential dangers such as insects, bees, the poison ivy plant, or the ragweed plant. After-school activities should not include painting, chalking, gluing, or plastic and rubber molding; it should rather consist of simple activities, such as music or stamp collecting.

Conclusion

Even though it is heartbreaking to see the atopic child singled out from his whole class, this will have less of an impact on him if his shortcomings are explained to him in a firm but nice way. Accepting his fate makes him less likely to suffer mental and physical anguish. All these restrictions, although hard to observe, help develop self-discipline in the child, and do not really deter him from achieving an education. Many children who have lived with handicaps have grown up to be successful in many fields of endeavor. What an atopic child needs most of all is an understanding mother and father, a loving family, some moral guidance, and a purpose in life. Other details in his upbringing are not that important because they come to him naturally, with a minimum of effort.

THE ENVIRONMENT OF THE ATOPIC CHILD AS A CAUSE OF OBSTRUCTIVE LUNG DISEASE

As a child ventures into the outside world, he leaves behind him the artificially created clean environment of his bedroom. Going to school, he must face the air of his city as it is, with its climatic features, its altitude, its temperature, as well as its barometric pressure changes. If his city lies at an altitude of six hundred feet or more above sea level, it may provide the child with little oxygen and create difficulty in breathing. On the other hand, if it has a dry and warm climate, it will permit the child to live outdoors and therefore catch fewer colds. If it is situated in a big industrial area, its air will be polluted, mixed with smoke, dust, odors, and exhaust gases from cars. This unclean air damages the nasal mucosa and its filtering hairs, which then fall off. This invariably leads to trouble because a child has to breathe thirty-five pounds of air daily, and with every breath he takes he is invaded by the great number of particles suspended in it. His nose is his first line of defense against these particles. Small hairs lining the nasal mucosa screen the particles out, catch them, mix them with its mucus, and expel them with a sneeze. If the inhaled particles are not expelled, they cause the mucosa to swell, become inflamed, and close up. It then requires the frequent use of nose drops to cause the mucosa to open up. Excessive use of nose drops causes a rebound effect and makes the situation worse. Rebound is a side effect of the protracted use of decongestants, which cause the nasal mucosa to swell, become more congested, and become refractory to further treatment. It is directly related to drug potency, and occurs with local as well as with systematic use of decongestants. The changes it brings about disturb the sense of smell of the child, who will not enjoy the odor of tasty food, or refuse that of spoiled food. At the same time, his stomach secretory reflex, which is activated by the smell of food, does not take place, and he will not feel like eating. Furthermore, chronic irritation in the nasal mucosa brings about polyp formation. Polyps will make the nose lose its resonance, become a trap for the bacteria of the sinuses, and hamper the free flow of air through the nostrils. They will force the child to breathe unmoisturized air through his mouth, directly into his lungs. This causes infections in the lungs, and creates chronic obstructive lung diseases.

To prevent damage to the hairs and mucosa of the nose through air impurities, the following measures are helpful:

1. A child going to school in a big city like New York or Yokohama should be made to wear a mask. If he is apprehensive about wearing the mask, one can advise a five-centimeter square of thin polyethylene to which is attached a thin strip of adhesive tape at its inner edge. The tape is applied to the upper lip, just below the nostrils, and the free edge of the strip is allowed to lie against the nostrils. The strip then exerts a valvular effect: it allows the air to go out, and moves up to close the nose when the child breathes in. The material is easily available, and sells under the name of "art foam." Such foam lets in clean air by filtering out all its impurities.

2. During the night, polluted air has to be cleaned with elaborate machinery placed in the bedroom. Two types of machines can be used for this purpose, a filtering devise or an electrostatic precipitator. The latter is the better one. It is a box that gives an electrical charge to the particles of dirt suspended in the air. The electrically charged particles are made to pass through a collection chamber, where another electrical charge makes them fall. They can be removed from the bottom of the box by cleaning it with water and detergent once a month.

If nothing succeeds, and the child has difficulty in breathing while going to school or while playing, we have to think of chronic obstructive lung diseases. These are a group of conditions that obstruct air flow within the lung. The group includes asthma, chronic bronchitis, pre-emphysema, emphysema and bronchiectasis. Asthma is characterized by episodic bronchospasm, usually related to allergy. Chronic bronchitis is excessive bronchial mucus and persistent cough caused by smoking, air pollution, repeated infections, or allergy. Pre-emphysema is an enlargement of the distal air spaces of the lungs, while emphysema is a destruction of the alveolar walls. Although these various disorders may coexist, pre-emphysema and emphysema are the only ones responsible for X-ray changes, abnormal blood gases, and difficult breathing with any slight effort.

Pre-Emphysema

This is a distension of the alveoli caused by air retention. Different from emphysema, a disease in which there is an irreversible breaking of the elastic fibers of the alveoli, pre-emphysema is a reversible and curable disease. Pre-emphysema may be prevented and treated as follows:

1. An asthmatic child who lives in a large city with polluted air is subject to frequent respiratory infections, which predispose him to pre-emphysema. He will do better in a small city in some place such as Arizona, Colorado, or California, where the air is relatively clean and warm, and where there are no great industries and few cars. In Europe, some very specialized places, like the underground caves of the Polish Salt Mines, may provide a temporary haven for a very sick child.

2. A child who has pre-emphysema must, since his back is made of bone and cannot stretch, be taught to use his abdominal muscles to press on his intestines during inspiration. The effort is transmitted toward his diaphragm and then to the base of his lungs, where it helps push out the stagnant air.

3. A child with pre-emphysema must be taught how to breathe through his nose only, because this warms, filters, and moisturizes the air. Also, he must be instructed not to fatigue himself while walking, exercising, pushing, lifting heavy weights, or doing physical work, because these activities increase his requirements for oxygen.

4. The following suggestions may improve pre-emphysema: (a) smoking must be prohibited in the house; (b) colds should be prevented and their complications treated with antibiotics; (c) a daily regime of bronchial hygiene consisting of opening up the airways with a bronchodilator aerosol, followed by inhalation of vapor to soften the mucus, plus breathing exercises, helps produce efficient expectoration of the mucus from the lungs.

5. The following breathing exercises are helpful: (a) while lying down and breathing correctly, a child should be able to move a ten-pound shot bag up and down on his abdomen without moving his chest; (b) while sitting up and leaning slightly forward, correct breathing should move the abdomen forward and back; (c) while standing and walking, correct breathing should be practiced in a slightly stooped position, with the weight on the soles of the feet.

Emphysema

A Historical Background to Emphysema

City air is stagnant, turbid and thick, the natural result of its big buildings, narrow streets and the refuse of its inhabitants. One should choose for a residence a wide-open site with ample sunshine and toilets located as far as possible from the living rooms. The air of the residence should be kept dry at all times by sweet scents, fumigation, and drying agents. Clean air plays the foremost role in preserving the health of one's body and soul.

—Written by Moses Maimonides in the year 1199

Emphysema is a disease caused by the breaking down of the elastic fibers of the lungs. The word is a Greek one, meaning "overinflation," that is, the lungs act like an overstretched spring that has lost its elasticity. They cannot expand to get fresh air, or recoil to expel stale air. To understand the analogy, one has to understand how the lungs work.

The lungs are made up of spongy, elastic tissue, hanging in sealed compartments in the chest. In normal breathing, when the muscles of the diaphragm and chest walls expand the size of the compartments, the lungs expand to fill them by filling themselves with air. When the muscles relax, the force of compression empties the lungs. An emphysematous lung can neither expand nor contract because its elastic tissue is destroyed. Its air sacs become bloated with air that gets trapped in them, and the lung looks like an over-inflated balloon.

In adults, the cause of emphysema is mainly smoking, while in children it may be caused by frequent upper respiratory infections, bronchial asthma, or air pollution. Air pollution is that state of the air in a big city which comes about when man-made wastes are produced so rapidly that they accumulate in concentrations that cannot be disposed of by the normal self-cleaning propensities of the atmosphere. Pollution consists of fog, dust, smoke, soot, sulfur dioxide, carbon monoxide, and carbon dioxide. At times, emphysema in a child may come about as a result of a "summation" effect of the above-mentioned three causes.

Diagnosis

Emphysema is a progressive disease that is difficult to diagnose in its earlier stages. Clinically, its most frequent sign is shortness of breath, a tendency to tire easily, weakness, coughing, wheezing, a feeling of tightness in the chest, and dizziness. None of these symptoms, however, is specific to emphysema, and pulmonary function tests are needed to make the exact diagnosis.

The Physiopathology of Emphysema

To understand the treatment of emphysema, we must first understand its physiopathology. In emphysema there is a loss of elasticity in the lungs that narrows their alveoli and promotes infections. Infections bring about a secretion of mucus and irritation. This irritation causes a muscular spasm in the bronchi, which in their turn become narrower. The narrowing of the bronchi impairs the free flow of air in between the lungs and body tissues, and causes a lack of oxygen and an abundance of carbon dioxide in the body tissues. The tissues fight off this condition by forming an excess of red blood cells to carry more of the needed oxygen and to remove the accumulated carbon dioxide. The excess of red blood cells hampers circulation, promotes clot formation, and fatigues the heart—which may cause it to fail. If it fails, the tissues will be supplied with even less oxygen, and have even more carbon dioxide. Retention of carbon dioxide by the tissues causes acidosis, a condition characterized by headaches, dehydration, malnutrition, personality changes, irrationality, emotional exhaustion, shock, and coma.

Treatment

There is no spontaneous recovery or known cure for emphysema. Its treatment aims at arresting its further progress, relieving its symptoms, and helping the patient achieve a more comfortable existence. It consists of a regime of breathing exercises, postural drainage exercises, avoidance of respiratory irritants, and aerosols. Aerosols are drugs reduced to very small particles and suspended in a gas that can be pushed forcefully into the lungs by means of a rubber hand bulb or an electric pump. A sophisticated machine used for this purpose is one called the *intermittent positive pressure machine,* or IPP. It can push antibiotics into the lungs to fight off an infection, bronchodilators to relax the muscles of the bronchi, enzymes to soften the mucus, and oxygen to ease cyanosis.

The most important chemical an emphysematous child may need is oxygen. Oxygen is a colorless gas that forms one-fifth of the volume of the air that a child breathes. It is essential to his respiration because it combines with other elements in the body to oxidize them. When oxidation occurs, light is generated, and a combustion takes place. This combustion is a source of energy. If there is not enough oxygen to carry out the combustion, there will be no energy to promote daily activities. The body will be in a semidormant state, in need of a supplement of oxygen. A supplement of oxygen may be given either with a mask, a nasal catheter, a tent, or an air chamber. Its concentration must be from 70 to 100 percent, and it must be adequately humidified.

An adequate oxygen supply for an emphysematous child is an extremely important part of his treatment; indeed, it forms the logical basis on which such treatment rests. We must guard, however, against excesses in oxygen therapy so we do not suppress the stimulus to respiration brought about by the presence of CO_2. Liquefying the mucus in the bronchi, fighting off the edema that forms there, controlling infection, and reducing the spasm of the muscles of the bronchi are nothing but steps aimed at opening up the bronchi to facilitate the free flow of oxygen through them.

The emphysematous child also has to be taught how to breathe efficiently to save oxygen. He must relax during inhalation to allow the abdomen to protrude and the diaphragm to descend, and he must breathe with pursed lips, taking three counts to breathe in and six or seven to breathe out. While walking, he must proceed as follows: He must inhale through his nose, because this warms, moisturizes, and filters the air he breathes. He must not get into the habit of taking extra deep breaths, because this fills the lungs with air, and he must not worry over the shortness of breath he experiences. (Shortness of breath in exercise is only an indication that the body needs more oxygen.) By slowing the rate of breathing, and concentrating on exhaling through pursed lips, one can spare oxygen and restore it to the system rapidly.

Emphysema, Pre-Emphysema, and the Asthmatic Child

An asthmatic child who suffers from these two diseases must avoid:

1. Smoke from cigarettes or charring food, extremes of temperature variation, wind, gassy or overripe foods or cold drinks.

2. Aerosol sprays of all types, from air fresheners and insecticides to deodorant and hair sprays.

3. Strong odors of all kinds: moth balls, colognes, perfumes, after-shave lotions, chlorine bleaches, smelly detergents.

4. Powders, such as bath powder, soap powders, and dusts.

5. The known allergens, whether they be inhalants (pollen, dust, or molds), or foods.

6. Aspirin and penicillin.

7. Respiratory infections (by not exposing himself to them and by using any required antibiotic quickly).

8. Overtreatment with steroids.

9. Strenuous exercises, stress (including that incurred by watching thriller TV shows), excessive sweating.

10. Going to zoos, movie houses, using moldy basements, or swimming in chlorinated pools.

Furthermore, the child or his parents must remember to discuss all physical or psychological problems freely with the child's physician, whether pertinent to his asthma or not. He must also remain indoors, as far as possible from automobile- and factory-congested areas, and keep quiet to reduce the volume of air breathed.

The child can also use on and off a new drug called Alupent which decreases the bronchial spasm usually associated with emphysema. It is a drug administered with a metered dose inhaler and can be used only by those children who are mature enough to grasp the significance of its side effects and its adverse reactions. These side effects and reactions are similar to those caused by all sympathomimetic agents, such as adrenalin or Iso. Two or three inhalations of the drug may give significant relief if given two or three times daily.

Fighting Air Pollution, Asthma, and Emphysema

All city residents must be made aware of the dangers of air pollution and should join one of these organizations:

Citizens for Clear Air, Inc.
502 Park Avenue
New York, N.Y. 10002

Citizens for a Quieter City
135 East 57th Street
New York, N.Y. 10019

Environment!
119 Fifth Avenue
New York, N.Y. 10003

Environmental Action Coalition
235 East 49th Street
New York, N.Y. 10017

NYS Action for Clean Air Committee
105 East 22nd Street
New York, N.Y. 10010

SUMMER VACATION AND CAMP

Summer is the time of the year when pollen and molds are present in the air in large quantities. Furthermore, it is camp time and outdoor time. Following are suggestions for "taming the outdoors" for the atopic child during a summer vacation.

Plan the child's vacations around his allergies; try not to leave one allergen behind, only to run into another one in the vacation area. Travel in an air-conditioned car, because car air-conditioning recirculates air and does not bring in outside air laden with allergens. While on his vacation, the child should wear light, solid colors, and not bright contrasting ones, and should avoid using sweetly scented hair preparations or tonics and anything else that would attract bees and insects. Also, going barefoot or wearing sandals invites stings. If needed, a fast-acting insecticide kept in a handy spot can be used to scatter bees and insects.

Pollen concentrations rise sharply close to their source, and one must cut down the ragweed near the vacation area to diminish this concentration. Also, plants discharge pollen primarily in the morning, and more intensely when the air is dry. Therefore, evenings and humid days are best for enjoying the outdoors of the vacation area. In that area, there should be no mowing of grass, in order not to churn up old mold spores, arouse bees and yellow jackets, or fill the air with pollen. Please note that:

1. A hedgerow or stand of trees can help reduce the amount of wind-blown pollens that enter the house; however, one must make sure that the windbreak itself doesn't cause allergies.

2. Make sure not to "freshen" the wash by hanging it out to dry. Damp clothing is a sure trap for airborne pollens.

3. Do not burn poison ivy plants, as smoke from burning poison ivy can cause extremely uncomfortable and potentially dangerous respiratory and skin irritations. It is better to spray the poison ivy plant to kill it and also to cut its stems close to the ground.

4. Avoid outdoor pets, because in addition to their own dander, they often carry lots of pollen in their coats, as well as poison ivy oil.

Many allergic children are sent to camp during the summer vacation, and in the United States many camps have been started that are pollen and mold free and serve hypoallergenic food. These camps keep the child all summer; he returns home at the end of the pollen and mold seasons. All the camps have a doctor on the premises who keeps a record of the specific allergies of the child, his blood type, his Rh factor, the dates of his immunizations, and the instructions for his desensitizing injections.

For information on nonprofit camps for children in the New York area refer to:

Community Council of Greater New York
225 Park Avenue South
New York, N.Y. 10003 (Tel. 212 775-5000); or

Association of Jewish Sponsored Camps, Inc.
130 East 59th Street
New York, N.Y. 10022 (Tel. 212 751-1000).

Before going to camp, the allergic child must be taught how to recognize and avoid bees, insects, the poison ivy leaf, and animals with furs or feathers. He must be given an emergency kit that contains antihistamines and Isuprel tablets, and be taught how to use them. He must be provided with light cotton clothing, and allergy-free soaps.

Once at camp, the child may swim in the ocean, but not in chlorinated pools. He may take long walks, but not in woods or infested areas. He must wear sunglasses to protect himself against strong sun rays, and use ultraviolet absorbing oils on his skin when he is outdoors for long periods of time. He must wear a tag indicating his drug, insect, or food allergies. These may be obtained as a bracelet or a metal medallion from Medic Alert Foundation, Turlock, Calif. 95380, or from National Identification Company, 3955 Oneida Street, Denver, Colo. 80207.

Improved health protection for children attending summer camps in New York State is provided in new regulations recently adopted by the State Public Health Council. Special requirements for children's camps include accident and fire prevention programs, the presence of at least one adult counselor for every eight children, and discontinued use by 1976 of nonfire-resistant buildings used for sleeping quarters by as many as thirty children or more.

A national listing of camps for asthmatic children, their capacity, and entrance requirements can be found on the following page. The end of this chapter can also be consulted for information on ragweed refuges in the United States, Canada, Bermuda, and Mexico.

Hay Fever

Outdoor living during the summer months exposes a child to pollen and molds and brings about hay fever. This is a seasonal disease, and every spring, summer, and fall about ten million children in the United States develop this illness. Although its name denotes an allergy to grasses, it is caused by numerous plants and also by many types of molds.

Hay fever begins after the age of three, and is equally distributed among boys and girls. The white race is more afflicted by it than

Camps for Asthmatic Children

LOCATION	NAME OF CAMP	MEDICAL DIRECTOR
CALIFORNIA Santa Cruz Mountains	Allergy Foundation of Northern California	Robert Dermott, M.D. 141 Camino Alto Mill Valley, Calif. 94941
KENTUCKY Lexington	Camp Weasel	Kenneth L. Gerson, M.D. University of Kentucky Medical Center Lexington, Ky. 40506
MINNESOTA Minneapolis	Camp Sdikrepus	Richard T. Cushing, M.D. 5000 West 39th Street Minneapolis, Minn. 55416
NEW YORK Adirondack Mountains	Camp Massawixie	Boy Scout Council of Monroe County 474 East Avenue Rochester, N.Y. 14607
Chappaqua	Wagon Road Camp	Armond V. Mascia, M.D. 200 South Broadway Tarrytown, N.Y. 10591
WASHINGTON Seattle	Children's Orthopedic Hospital & Medical Center Camp	S. J. Stamm, M.D. 4800 Sandpoint Way, N.E. Seattle, Wash. 98105
WEST VIRGINIA Red House (25168) R.D. #1	Bronco Junction	Merle S. Scherr, M.D. 805 Atlas Building Charleston, W. Va. 25301

AREA SERVED		BED CAPACITY		AGE		LENGTH OF STAY		
Local	Out of State	Total	Asthma	Min.	Max.	Min.	Avg.	Max.
Yes	No	50	50	8	14		1 wks.	
Yes	No	50	50	7	16		2 wks.	
Yes	No	80	80	6	15		2 wks.	
Yes	No							
Yes	No	80	30	8	15	3 wks.		6 wks.
Yes	NW	125	50	5			5 days	
Yes	Yes	60	60	6	16	8 wks.	8 wks.	8 wks.

the black and yellow races, while the American Indian does not have it at all. It is found all over the globe, but it is most prevalent in the temperate zone.

The symptoms of hay fever begin in the early hours of the morning with acute attacks of sneezing, nasal obstruction, profuse watery discharge from the nose, and itching and watering of the eyes. Some minor symptoms, such as a buzzing sensation in the ear, a dry irritating cough, headaches, slight temperature elevation, and nervousness may also be present. However, certain substances may cause symptoms similar to those of hay fever. These are: dust, cosmetics, chemical fumes, strong light rays, tobacco smoke, and chlorine in swimming pools.

The diagnosis of hay fever is usually easy because the disease follows a strictly seasonal course.

Knowledge about the pollen of the plants and the spores of the molds that cause hay fever is important because no hay fever diagnosis is complete and exact unless the incidence in the air of the implicated pollen or mold matches the results of the skin tests and the clinical course of the disease.

Pollen As a Cause of Hay Fever

Pollen is the male element of a flower. It can do its fertilizing job only if it is carried from one flower to another by bees or the wind. Not all pollen is allergenic. Allergenic pollen usually comes from small flowers that have no scent or nectar, and therefore do not attract bees, and are found in large quantities around inhabited areas. The pollen of these flowers is carried by the wind, which is what causes it to be dangerous. The pollen of large and colorful flowers causes no allergies because such flowers attract bees; the pollen therefore does not float freely in the air but sticks inadvertently to the bodies of the bees, and does its fertilizing job as the bees hop from one flower to another.

Certain trees, grasses, and weeds have highly allergenic pollen. In the United States the following trees produce it: oak, poplar, beech, elm, hickory, ash, birch, and maple. These are all common trees, found in many back yards or planted along streets, and they flower for a few days in April or in May. However, their importance in the overall picture of pollen allergy is minimal, because only 10 percent of pollen-sensitive children suffer from allergy to tree pollen. Even then, recognizing these trees is important; they may have to be removed from the yard of a child who is sensitive to them.

Grasses are more important than trees in causing pollen sensitivity. For each child who is sensitive to tree pollen there are three who are sensitive to grass pollen. Grasses are found in lawns and meadows all over the world and in all climates, but they thrive best in the temperate zone. In the United States, grasses pollinate from May until August; in Europe, grasses usually pollinate earlier and die earlier, while in some temperate zones, such as Israel, they remain in active pollination for eight months of the year. Unlike the trees, which in pollen-sensitivity tests have to be considered on an individual basis, almost any one grass may be taken and used indiscriminately in testing for all grasses, or in their treatment. There are only a few exceptions to this rule, and these exceptions do not change the overall picture.

The most important cause of weed pollen allergy in the United States is the pollen of the ragweed plant. Two out of every three pollen-sensitive children are allergic to it. There is a short variety of ragweed, a tall variety, and a giant one, but they all cause the same type of allergy. They start pollinating around August 15 and continue to do so until the first frost. All weeds are extremely strong plants; they can live in poor soil and under severe weather conditions, but they cannot survive frost.

Molds As a Cause of Hay Fever

Many children with hay fever find that on occasion they suffer more discomfort than they expected on days when the pollen count is relatively low. This is a clue that the child may be suffering from an additional allergy, probably a sensitivity to molds.

Molds belong to the family of plants known as fungi. Some types are well known because they are used in the manufacture of antibiotics, such as penicillin and streptomycin. The molds that cause trouble are of a different type. They are primitive plants that have no roots, stems, or leaves, and that sporulate in the summer months, causing allergies then. They procure their food from dead plants, from leaves, or from rotting vegetables and fruits. They act as scavengers of the soil, and convert the dead material they eat into fertilizer. A mold consists of a "root," which is embedded in the soil, and a body of thin threads that goes up in the air and bears a fruit called a *spore*. The spore gets detached from the threads of the mold, is carried away in the air, lands on an adjacent soil, and becomes another mold. While in the air, it may act as an inhalant, and cause allergies in the same way that pollen does, that is, it sensitizes by merely being present in the air.

Molds live best at 70 to 90°F.; they stop growing about 40°F. They are able to survive freezing for months, but they do not survive high temperatures; they die around the boiling point. They live in a mother dwelling, but their spores can be scattered around for many miles during a storm. Different locales have different types of molds, and each locale needs its own mold survey. Although the outside molds are the important ones, some molds that manage to grow in old furniture and in damp basements cause trouble too. A survey of these molds should be done by culturing them in appropriate media. This information may be used later in the desensitization program.

Although there are more than fifty thousand species of fungi, certain ones seem to be the main offenders. Alternaria, one of the most prevalent, is considered to be the prime troublemaker, followed by hormodendrum, penicillium, and aspergillus.

Allergy to molds is not sharply seasonal, as is pollen allergy. As the warm weather approaches, the mold spore count rises but not in any predictable manner. Damp, humid and hot weather is favorable for their dispersal.

One peculiarity of mold allergy is its absence when snow is on the ground (snow does not permit the spores to leave the ground).

Another peculiarity is its connection with mold-containing foods, such as Roquefort and Camembert cheeses, beer, and Chinese sauces. A third peculiarity is its frequency among farmers who handle manure, compost, or dead leaves in barns.

The diagnosis of mold allergy is done by taking an allergic history, and then performing intracutaneous tests. Scratch tests are not to be used for molds. The reading of the tests is done after fifteen minutes, but molds may give delayed reactions after a day or two.

The prevention of mold allergy consists of avoiding seashores, barns, and wooded areas; using a Dacron-filled sleeping bag when camping; removing fallen leaves and damp grass from the back yard; washing the tiles and grout of the bathroom; checking stored food for spoilage; exposing damp shoes, boots, or sneakers to the sun; avoiding indoor plants and dried flowers; venting the clothes dryer, and checking all humidifiers, dehumidifiers, and air-conditioners for musty smells; throwing away all old and damp furniture.

Basements suspected of harboring molds have to be sanitized with detergents, drying agents, and electrostatic precipitators. Some chemicals check mold growth, and these are available through the following sources:

Allergy Free Products for the Home
P.O. Box 345, 1162 West Lynn Street
Springfield, Mo. 65801; or

Fleming and Company
9730 Reavis Park Drive
St. Louis, Mo. 63123.

Complications of Hay Fever

Untreated hay fever may turn into asthma; it may cause frequent infections in the nose and sinuses, the formation of polyps in the nose, nosebleeds, loss of smell, inflammation in the eyes, dizziness, mental disturbances, slight temperature elevation, vernal conjunctivitis and hearing loss.

Vernal conjunctivitis is an allergic disease that is frequently seen among male children in warm climates. It occurs during the spring and early summer and continues on and off until the beginning of winter. It manifests itself in two ways. One involves the eyelid and its conjunctive, and the other the cornea. The lid type develops a characteristic cobblestone appearance, and secretes a thick, ropy material. The corneal, or limbic, type is characterized by small vesicles that appear at the rim of the cornea. The cause of the disease is probably an allergic reaction of the conjunctiva or cornea to heat and light. Its symptoms are a fear of light (photophobia), tearing, a burning sensation in the eyes, some itching, and a foreign body sensation in the eye. Its diagnosis is made by its seasonal occurrences, and the cobblestone picture of the conjunctiva. The condition has to be differentiated from other allergic manifestations in the eye caused by drugs, cosmetics, soaps, inhalant allergens, nonspecific eye irritants (polluted air), bacteria, and foods. Its treatment consists of corticosteroid drops put locally (1 drop of 1 percent hydrocortisone solution) three to four times daily for one or two weeks. If this is not sufficient, corticosteroids have to be given by mouth.

Hearing Loss

Hearing loss caused by allergy is frequently detected in school through a routine audiogram. The events that bring about this partial deafness in one or both ears start with edema and blockage of the eustachian tubes. This causes an absorption of the air present in the middle ear and a drop in its pressure. Low pressure brings about an oozing of fluid in the middle ear chamber, a condition called *serous otitis media*. If this fluid thickens, it becomes mucoid, and gets secondarily infected. It causes a hearing loss, a sense of fullness in the ears, ringing sounds, and giddiness. If this fluid remains in the middle ear for two to three months, its pressure on the inner ear will cause deafness.

Although the immediate cause of blockage in the eustachian

tubes is edema brought about by an allergy to pollen, molds, dust, or foods, congenital defects in the tubes proper or the arches of the palate that surround them, may predispose the child to this condition and precipitate it.

The treatment of this condition consists of ventilation of the middle ear through decongestants and antihistamines; eradication of infection with antibiotics; removal of the middle ear fluid; removal of enlarged tonsils and adenoids that may be mechanically blocking the fluid drainage; control of allergies through diet, environmental control, desensitization, upper respiratory vaccines, gamma globulins, and corticosteroids.

Symptomatic Treatment of Hay Fever

This consists of avoiding the allergen (pollen or mold), taking medication for the relief of symptoms, and desensitization (see page 117). Avoidance of the allergen while in the bedroom can be accomplished by means of filtration through Hepa Filters or electrostatic precipitation, while its avoidance in the area is done through a vacation in a pollen- and mold-free resort. The drugs that give symptomatic relief are divided into two categories: the antihistamines and the steroids. Antihistamines give relief by drying up the secretions of the nose, and by providing general tranquilization. The steroids are potent anti-inflammatory drugs, which work through the mobilization or substitution of the body hormone reserve. Neither prevents hay fever in future years.

Pollen and Mold-free Areas

For those who suffer from hay fever, accurate advice about ragweed and mold air pollution in the various parts of the country is of great importance. Following is a state by state list for the United States and Canada on air contamination caused by ragweed. Since some areas are changing rapidly, names of all places may not be given here. Parents should contact their local medical society for the names of cities and places that are not supplied. The term "excellent" is used to denote a perfect locality, "good" to denote a place where most children will have relief, and "not recommended" to denote places that should be avoided. The mold-free areas are listed below.

Ragweed Pollen Refuges in the U.S.A. and Its Island Territories

Alabama. The Gulf Coast at Foley, good (nine consecutive seasons); fairly good at Mobile (three seasons). Field surveys throughout the remainder of the state reveal wide distribution of ragweed in waste places and on farms. Birmingham has a very poor record.

Alaska. No ragweed pollen was found as a result of atmospheric tests made in three places (Nome, Fairbanks, and Juneau) for one season.

Arizona. Excellent rating for the north and south rims of Grand Canyon. During the fall season in Phoenix conditions are excellent, but there is a spring ragweed season of at least moderate consequence. Our best information for the Tucson area gives it a rating of good for both spring and fall. For other communities in the state there are no atmospheric data.

Arkansas. The average exposure to ragweed pollen throughout the state is doubtless very heavy. No refuge areas are known.

California. *Excellent:* Lassen Volcanic National Park, Sequoia National Park, Oakland, Sacramento, San Francisco, Monterey, Yountville, Yosemite National Park, Los Angeles, Pasadena, El Centro, Escondido, San Diego, Tujunga.
    Good: Alpine, Arcata, Santa Barbara.
    While air sampling has not been done in the great central valley, it is unlikely that any community there or elsewhere in the state will be found to have an appreciable degree of ragweed pollen pollution.

Colorado. *Excellent:* Rocky Mountain National Park at Estes Park and Grand Lake, Mesa Verde National Park, Glenwood Springs, the crest of Pike's Peak.

Good: Colorado Springs. Formerly this city's record was not so good. Ragweed is not common on the west of the slope; sagebrush is likely to be encountered in this area. Close exposure should be avoided by ragweed-sensitive persons.

Denver and the eastern third of the state constitute an area of moderate to heavy ragweed exposure.

Connecticut. Atmospheric studies have been made in eight cities. No refuge areas are known.

Delaware. Field studies show ragweed to be abundant throughout. Nearest atmospheric studies are those made at Philadelphia and Baltimore. No refuge areas are known.

District of Columbia and adjacent areas of Maryland show heavy ragweed pollen incidence.

Florida. *Excellent:* Santa Rosa Island, Key West, Fort Myers, Miami Beach, Coral Gables, Miami, Sunnyside Beach (Panama City).

Good: Daytona Beach, Orlando, Sebring, Bradenton, Everglades National Park, St. Petersburg, Fort Pierce, Live Oak, West Palm Beach.

Fairly good: Fort Lauderdale (Beach), Jacksonville, Tallahassee, Tampa, Clearwater, Pensacola.

Not recommended: Ocala, Gainesville, Melbourne, Panama City.

The beaches of Florida are almost uniformly desirable; inland areas are often not so good.

Georgia. Valdosta (only one season) fairly good. Central and northern Georgia and the coastal area, as judged by tests at Atlanta and St. Simon Island and as checked by widely scattered field surveys, have moderately heavy exposure. No recent data.

Hawaii. No significant amounts of any kind of ragweed have been found anywhere on the larger islands except in the area between Schofield Barracks and Pearl Harbor on Oahu. Honolulu is probably ragweed-pollen free on account of prevailing northeast trade winds. No daily atmospheric tests have ever been reported.

Idaho. *Excellent:* Sun Valley (two years), Moscow (one year).
Good: Boise, Pocatello.

All mountainous areas are likely excellent, but exposure to sagebrush pollen is possible throughout most of the state. Close contact with sagebrush should be strictly avoided.

Illinois. No refuge area. Heavy records in seventeen cities and towns.

Indiana. No refuge area. Heavy records in seven cities and towns.

Iowa. No refuge area. Heavy records in six cities and towns.

Kansas. No refuge area. Atmospheric ragweed pollen incidence diminishes westward.

Kentucky. No refuge areas are known, but are barely possible in the Cumberland Mountains.

Louisiana. Heavy atmospheric pollution at New Orleans. Air sampling has been carried on only at New Orleans and at Vicksburg, Mississippi, across the river from Tallulah, Louisiana. No recent reports.

Maine. *Excellent:* St. Francis, Greenville Junction, Millinocket, Presque Isle, Macwahoc, Quoddy Head, New Portland, Newagen, Enfield, Deblois, Belfast, Allagash, Grand Lake Stream, Bethel, Eagle Lake, Lincoln, Oquossoc, Speckle Mountain, Upper Dam.
Good: Houlton, Newport, Jackman, Machias, Bar Harbor, Boothbay Harbor.
Fairly good: Eastport, Rockland, Southport, York, Augusta, Camden, Rangeley, North Augusta, Orono.

Not recommended: Stonington, Poland Spring, Auburn, Alfred, Portland, Kineo.

Maryland. No refuge area is known. No atmospheric studies have been made in the mountainous parts of western Maryland.

Massachusetts. *Good:* Annisquam, East Gloucester, West Gloucester, Magnolia, Rockport, Nantucket Island.

Fairly good: Gloucester, Worcester.

Not recommended: Winchester, Boston, Northampton, Amherst, Newton Center.

This is the state, and Boston the chief city, from which ragweed hay fever victims first fled to the mountains and rocky coastal areas of New Hampshire and Maine some one hundred years ago. Even so, ragweed pollen is much less abundant in the air in Boston than in most of the larger cities of the northeastern United States. Of the fourteen communities tested, none offers excellent refuge conditions. Neither the Berkshires nor Cape Cod has received attention. Weed destruction seems to be effective on Nantucket Island. Otherwise ragweed takes over all waste areas.

Michigan. *Excellent:* Isle Royale National Park.

Good: Sault Ste. Marie, Copper Harbor.

Fairly good: Houghton.

Fifty years ago much of the area of northern Michigan was doubtless entirely free from ragweed and ragweed pollen, but sampling done in fifty-seven systematically selected communities during the past twenty-five years has shown that no effective refuges remain in the lower peninsula, and that those of the northern peninsula are few, as listed above. The following list does not include any city of the lower peninsula. Those toward the beginning of the list are much better than those toward the end and might be suitable for persons with moderate sensitivity.

Not recommended (upper peninsula only): Saint Ignace, Blaney, Munising, Ironwood, Mackinac Island, Newberry, Powers, Menominee, Escanaba.

Minnesota. *Fairly good:* Tower, Virginia. Other places as good as or better than Tower and Virginia could likely be found in other parts of the Arrowhead County (northeastern corner of the state).

Not recommended: Duluth, Rochester, Minneapolis, Winona, Moorhead. The state has been inadequately covered.

Mississippi. Biloxi, on the coast, is fairly good. Field studies reveal an abundance of ragweed on farms throughout, so except for the immediate coast no refuge areas are likely to be found.

Missouri. No refuge areas.

Montana. *Excellent:* Glacier National Park at Belton and Many Glacier, West Yellowstone. Judging by the excellent records for more than twenty cities and towns in the adjacent parts of Alberta and Saskatchewan and at Yellowstone National Park, most of Montana is practically free of ragweed.

Good: Miles City.

Very meager data and no recent studies for this state. Sagebrush is widely distributed and should be avoided by persons known to be ragweed sensitive.

Nebraska. No refuge areas, but considerably less ragweed is found in the western third of the state than in the eastern part.

Nevada. Very meager data, and no recent air sampling. Ragweed is rare along the principal highways. Reno, excellent. Lake Mead, excellent in the fall, good in the spring ragweed season. Sagebrush is a possible factor.

New Hampshire. *Excellent:* Moosilauke, Pawtuckaway, Errol, Lancaster, Carroll, Laconia, Colebrook, Blue Job Mountain, Derby, Groveton, Lincoln, Pittsburgh, Warren, Whitefield.

Good: Bath, Conway, Dixville, Littleton, North Conway, Ossipee, Hampton, Plymouth, Bethlehem, Crotched Mountain, Dover, Franklin, Hillsboro, Holderness, New London.

Fairly good: Claremont, Concord, Federal Hill, Keene, Berlin, New Ipswich, Manchester, Weirs.

Not recommended: Hinsdale, Charlestown, Rye, Rochester, Lebanon, Jeremy, Exeter, Peterboro, Nashua.

New Jersey. No refuge areas known. Those places along the northern shore where relief is sometimes found are subject to high counts when the wind blows from the west. Studies have been made in twenty-nine cities.

New Mexico. Very meager atmospheric data. Ragweed is probably comparatively rare throughout the state. Roswell is good, and Albuquerque fairly good.

New York. The reports on Long Island have produced variable records. Fire Island at Ocean Beach is sometimes fairly good, and Montauk likewise fairly good. No other records are available for the Island except in Brooklyn, which is not recommended.

Adirondack Area. *Excellent:* Keene Valley.
Good: Blue Mountain Lake, Elk Lake, Keene, Loon Lake.
Fairly good: Big Moose, Chilson, Indian Lake, Long Lake, McColloms, Raquette Lake, Paul Smiths, Redford, Wanakena, Chateaugay Lake, Inlet, Sabattis, Schroon Lake (Severance), Tupper Lake, Newcomb, Owl's Head, Lake Placid, McKeever.

Catskill Area. *Good:* Big Indian, Haines Falls, Pine Hill.
Fairly good: Fleischmanns.
Studies have been made in eighty-five other counties and communities, including all of the larger cities, none of which can be recommended.

North Carolina. No refuge areas are known, but air tests at Newfound Gap, Tennessee, on the crest of the Great Smoky Mountains prove the immediate area to be good. Most likely, there are other places equally good at similar or higher elevations in North Carolina. (No accommodations at Newfound Gap in the national park.) There are records of heavy concentration of ragweed pollen for four of the large cities in the state.

North Dakota. No atmospheric data are available except in the narrow Red River Valley at Fargo. No refuge areas are known, but conditions are likely to be much the same in the southern half of the state as in South Dakota. Judging from data available from adjacent areas in Canada, there might be some good places found along the north edge of the state.

Ohio. No refuge areas. Adequate sampling has been done in 7 large cities.

Oklahoma. No refuge areas. Adequate sampling has been done in 7 large cities.

Oregon. *Excellent:* Coquille, Corvallis, Eugene, Crater Lake National Park, Portland, Turner.

No atmospheric data studies have been made in eastern Oregon except at Milton-Freewater, which is good.

Pennsylvania. No refuge areas are known. Claims for mountain resorts have never been proven. Sampling has been carried on in ten large cities for many years.

Puerto Rico. No atmospheric studies have ever been reported, but recent careful examination failed to disclose any ragweed on the island.

Rhode Island. No refuge areas.

South Carolina. No refuge areas are known, but our data are very meager. Nothing recent.

South Dakota. There are no refuge areas better than fairly good (Rapid City, Mobridge).

Tennessee. No refuge areas are known. Along the crest of the Great Smoky Mountains at Newfound Gap conditions were found to be good. There are no accommodations at this point, but there might be places with similar conditions at similar or higher elevations.

Texas. Big Spring is the only community out of the ten where studies have been made that has a rating of good. Most of Texas is badly infested with ragweed. However, they diminish considerably toward the western corner of the state, for example in El Paso.

Utah. *Excellent:* Zion National Park, Bryce Canyon National Park.

Fairly good: Vernal in the extreme northeast corner of the state and Hurricane in the extreme southwest corner of the state.

The average for metropolitan Salt Lake City is fairly good, except for the Canyon Rim area.

Vermont. Very meager data. Conditions on the east side of the state are probably comparable to adjacent areas of New Hampshire. Heavy atmospheric contamination is found in the upper Lake Champlain area.

Virginia. No excellent or good refuge areas are known.

Virgin Islands. *Excellent:* The island of St. John (Virgin Islands National Park), the island of St. Thomas.

Washington. *Excellent:* Seattle-Tacoma Airport, Mt. Rainier National Park (Longmire, White River, Paradise Valley), Seattle, Olympic National Park, Spokane, Yakima.

Good: Walla Walla.

Except for the badly ragweed-contaminated orchards in the immediate vicinity of Wenatchee, all but one place among the ten tested in the state are excellent or good.

West Virginia. No refuge areas are known.

Wisconsin. No refuge areas are known, but no adequate investigation had been made in the vast lake region of the northern part of the state.

Wyoming. Very meager data except at the national parks.

Grand Teton National Park and Yellowstone National Park are excellent; Lander is not recommended.

Refuges in Canada

Alberta. With atmospheric tests in fourteen communities, we have the following report:

Excellent: Banff, Beaver Lodge, Edmonton, Jasper, Vermilion, Lake Louise, Cypress Hills, Waterton Lakes Park, Calgary, Coleman, Manyberries, Drumheller, Lethbridge.

Fairly good: Medicine Hat.

Sagebrush pollen is a possible irritant to ragweed sufferers in those parts of Alberta which have been covered by the surveys.

British Columbia. Meager data.

Excellent: Summerland, Saanichton, Victoria.

Manitoba. *Excellent:* The Pas, Riding Mountain National Park, Russell, Brandon.

Good: Dauphin.

Fairly good: Pierson, Winnipeg.

Sagebrush pollen is a possible irritant to ragweed sufferers in those parts of Manitoba which have been covered by the surveys.

New Brunswick. *Excellent:* Campbellton, Bathurst, Richibucto, Newcastle-Chatam, Dalhousie, Fredericton, Woodstock, Doaktown, McAdam, Shediac Cape, St. John, Grand Manan, Edmundston, Perth-Andover, St. George, Welsford, St. Andrews, St. Stephen, Chipman, Moncton, Sackville, Tracadie.

Good: Sussex, Haslam, Farm (Fundy National Park), Lakeview, Jemseg, Waterside (Fundy National Park).

Fairly good: Pointe du Chene, Gagetown.

No high concentrations were found at any place.

Newfoundland. Only two communities (Corner Brook, St. John's) on the island have been studied, and they are both excellent.

Nova Scotia. *Excellent:* Truro, Middle West Pubnico, Cape Breton, Highlands National Park, Chester, Antigonish, Baddeck, Igonish Island.

Good: Mateghan, Digby, Yarmouth, Kentville.
No other studies have been reported.

Ontario. Systematic atmospheric pollen research has been carried on in Ontario since 1928, gradually increasing in volume until records are now available for at least one season in seventy communities. For some communities there are now continuous annual records for more than thirty years. The well-populated area of southern Ontario from Windsor to Cornwall is about as heavily contaminated with ragweed as are the adjacent areas of less intensive cultivation or none at all, where ragweed pollution drops rapidly to insignificant levels.

Excellent: Timmins, Fort William, New Liskeard, Kapuskasing, Port Arthur, Fort Francis, Barry's Bay, Black Sturgeon Lake, Chalk River, Cochrane, South River, Haleburton.

Good: Blind River, Mattawa, Timagami, Lake Joseph, Magnetawan, Rosseau, Sudbury, Espanola, Muskata Falls, Tobermory.

Fairly good: Cedar Lake, Dorset, Pembroke, Renfrew, Sault Ste. Marie, Honey Harbor, Bancroft, Kenora, Mindemoya (Manitoulin Island), North Bay, Westport, Port Carlings.

Not recommended, at least for severe cases, in order of their degree of ragweed pollution from least to greatest: Huntsville, Smith Falls, Algonquin Park, Georgian Bay Islands National Park, Gravenhurst, Lion's Head, Ottawa, Parry South, Madoc, Wiarton, Cornwall, Kincardine, Point Pelee National Park, Bellville, Peterborough, Picton, St. Lawrence Islands National Park, London, Mallorytown, Toronto and metropolitan area, Windsor, Hamilton.

Prince Edward Island. *Excellent:* Cavendish Montague, Souris, Summerside, Tignish, Charlottetown, O'Leary.

Good: Prince Edward Island National Park.
No other studies have been reported.

Quebec. *Excellent:* Chandler, Iles de la Madeleine, Matapedia, Mont-Albert Caspesie, Gaspe, Grande Rivière, Mont Joli, Father Point, Carleton, Charlesburg, Percé, Tadoussac.

Good: Matane, New Carlisle, Normandin, Baie Saint-Paul, Jonquière (Chicoutimi), Lennoxville, St. Lambert.

Fairly good: St. Jovite, Lac des Plages, Mont Laurier, Nominingue, Mont Tremblant, Rimouski, Rivière du Loup, Ste. Anne de la Pocatière, Ste. Agathe, Lac des Seize Iles.

In the southwest tip of the province, adjacent to New York and New Hampshire, contamination is bad. North of the Ottawa and St. Lawrence Rivers, and in the Gaspe country, conditions are good to excellent.

Saskatchewan. *Excellent:* Prince Albert National Park, Nelford, Prince Albert, Scott, Regina, Saskatoon, Swift Current.

Other Areas Adjacent to the U.S.

Bermuda

Atmospheric tests have been made only at Hamilton, where no ragweed pollen was detected.

Cuba

Field inspection reveals a number of areas where common ragweeds grow along the roadsides, but the atmospheric tests reported from Havana give the city a rating of excellent.

Mexico

Good: Mexico City, Tampico, Torreon.

Not recommended: Ciudad Juarez, Matamoros.

Slender false ragweed and western ragweed are found in small amounts in all states as far south as Mexico City. Our best information is that ragweed pollen concentrations are very low in most parts and absent in the southern states.

Specific Treatment of Hay Fever and Other Allergies Through Skin Testing Followed by Desensitization

Skin Testing

Skin testing for inhalants, foods, and contactants is the introduction inside the layers of the skin of a minute quantity of an allergen. There are three methods used in skin testing. One is to scratch the surface of the skin and then to add an allergenic extract to the scratch; the second is to introduce, with a needle, a small quantity of an allergenic extract inside the layers of the skin. The first method is called the scratch test; the second the intracutaneous test. Fewer side effects occur with the scratch test, but the intracutaneous test is more effective and sensitive. The third method is patch testing. This is used to determine the cause of a contact dermatitis. It is a delayed type of reaction, which appears one or two days after the performance of the test. This contrasts with the immediate type of reaction in tests for foods and inhalants that appears only fifteen to thirty minutes after the test. A patch test consists of reproducing the disease by putting the suspected material in direct contact with the skin.

The interpretation of a skin test is difficult because a positive reaction in testing is not conclusive evidence of allergy unless it is confirmed by a history of allergic manifestations. A positive reaction may mean one of the following: a current allergy to the substance; a past allergy to the substance; a false allergy caused by a sensitivity to a substance similar to the testing substance; or a healthy child with an unexplained skin allergy.

Skin testing is an extremely valuable tool to identify inhalant allergens. By inhalant we mean one of the light allergens that float freely in the air, such as pollen, molds, animal dander, or bedroom incidentals. Skin testing, however, has shortcomings in detecting food allergies.

Desensitization

By desensitization is meant the giving of a series of injections of an allergen in increasing doses to diminish the sensitivity to that allergen. Indications that a sensitivity requires desensitization are (1) allergic symptoms that have been present for over three weeks during a particular season and that have required daily medication; (2) bronchial asthma that has occurred during the period of pollination of a pollen or the sporulation of a mold; (3) the concomitant occurrence of symptoms in more than one organ; for example, in the eye and nose; (4) a strongly positive intracutaneous skin test.

When the skin tests are completed, a child with hay fever is classified into one of five categories: AA, A, B, C, and D, depending on the intensity of his skin reaction to the allergen. Injection treatment then follows, and this is based on the degree of sensitivity of the child to each single allergen.

In desensitization treatment, we may use one of three methods: (1) a co-seasonal one, that is, starting injections during the season of the pollen in question; (2) a preseasonal one, that is, starting injections three months before the season; or (3) a perennial one, that is, giving injections throughout the year. The last is the type of desensitization used by the majority of allergists. At the beginning, the child receives one injection weekly, and once the maximum tolerated dose is reached after four or five months, the frequency is slowly reduced to one injection per month. Injections are to be given for three or four consecutive years, and when the child is symptom free for two years desensitization treatment is stopped.

Minor colds and slight allergic symptoms are not reasons for missing injections, but major illnesses must postpone treatment.

Aqueous extracts of allergens, oily extracts of allergens, pyridine-precipitated extracts of allergens, alum-precipitated extracts of allergens, and detoxified extracts of allergens are all used in desensitization. Aqueous extracts, however, are considered to be the best desensitizing agents, and all rational treatment of allergies today rests on their usage. Pyridine-precipitated extracts are not solutions but suspension of allergens. With these extracts, fewer injections are needed for hyposensitization, the local and constitutional reactions are fewer, highly allergic children tolerate them better, and they are more economical. However, a final verdict on their efficiency has not been passed yet by the great majority of allergists. Alum-precipitated extracts are new and the author has had no experience with them. Extracts of allergens in mineral oil (the one-shot treatment) has practically gone out of use, and detoxified extracts await further studies.

Two types of reactions may occur when a child receives a desensitizing injection: a local reaction in the place of the injection, or a generalized systemic reaction. If proper care is taken in giving the injection, the dangers of a reaction are reduced to a minimum. A child who has received an injection should remain in the doctor's office for twenty minutes after the injection, and should be seen by the physician before he leaves. It is not wise, however, to give him antihistamines before the injections in the hope of avoiding reactions. Antihistamine may obscure mild symptoms, but open the way for dangerous systemic reactions with a future injection.

Any injection that has caused a local reaction that lasted twelve hours or more should be repeated in future administrations until there are no more local reactions. If the local reaction lasts for forty-eight hours, then the dose should be reduced to the one that did not cause any reaction. Any injection that has given a systemic reaction (sneezing, coughing, wheezing, hives, or anaphylactic shock) must be judged according to its severity. Discontinuance of therapy should be the rule if anaphylaxis has occurred even with a small dose. Systemic reactions are usually caused by giving a larger dose than the child can tolerate, by increasing a dosage from a concentrated vial instead of a previously used, less concentrated vial, by making a mistake in the dosage of the injection, by accidental intravenous injection, and by changing from one year's extract to the next without having properly reduced the dosage. (Desensitizing injections are biological extracts that deteriorate on keeping.) The treatment of systemic reactions consists of the following measures:

For mild reactions, place a tourniquet above the site of the injection; inject 0.3 cc. adrenalin in the area of the injection; give antihistamines by mouth. For moderate reactions (hives, laryngeal edema, asthma), give an injection of adrenalin and oxygen by inhalation if there is cyanosis; hospitalize for possible tracheotomy.

For severe reactions (an anaphylactic shock), give adrenalin, oxygen, and intravenous fluids, preferably in a hospital.

There is no use in desensitizing against foods or certain animals. However, desensitization against pollen and dust gives significant relief to 80 percent of the children who have it over a period of three to four years. Desensitization against molds is very difficult to handle, and the results of this treatment are unpredictable. Lastly, desensitization against bacteria using stock vaccines is hard to evaluate, but autogenous vaccines taken from the *inside* of the tonsils and adenoids of the child sometimes give good results.

A desensitization treatment may fail because it may not have been indicated, because the solution may not have been prepared by a reputable firm, because local reactions may not have been accounted for, because the allergens were not eliminated completely from the environment, or because some children have a positive skin reaction to an allergen without being sensitive to it.

A Case History: Reaction to Desensitization
Subject: D.S.
Age: 5 years
Symptoms: D.S. was being treated for grass pollen allergy with weekly injections. In the course of his treatment, the allergist switched from one desensitizing bottle to a more concentrated bottle while still giving the boy the right amount of pollen. Twenty minutes after the injection, D.S.'s eyes became congested, his face got red, and a rash developed over his body. The allergist injected ⅓ cc. of adrenalin in the site of the injection, and gave him antihistamines by mouth. The symptoms disappeared in half an hour.
Comments: D.S.'s reaction was caused by the fact that the second bottle of extract was relatively more potent than the first one. Pollen extracts lose some potency when kept for some time. Also, the same pharmaceutical house may prepare two batches of the same extract that may differ slightly in their potency; furthermore, batches prepared by different houses may differ substantially in their potency. We are dealing with a biological extract and not with a stable chemical solution.

7 Bronchial Asthma in Babies and Children

AN INTRODUCTION TO ASTHMA

In normal breathing the lungs inhale fresh air and expel stale air without effort. This is done through a system of branching tubes, which end up in a sac with very thin walls. Through these walls, oxygen and carbon dioxide from the blood vessels that surround the sac go in and out of it in opposite directions to fuel the cells of the body, or to remove its waste products. Allergy, air pollution, and respiratory infections may turn easy breathing into a difficult process called asthma.

Asthma is a general term to denote any disease that is characterized by attacks of difficult breathing and wheezing sounds in the chest. These attacks may subside in a few minutes or last for a few days, and have a behavior that is totally unpredictable: they may appear at any age; they may develop suddenly or gradually; they may disappear for no reason, reappear or become chronic.

The characteristics of asthma in a child are different from those of an adult:

1. In the child, asthma tends to be related to specific allergens, is usually atopic and hereditary, begins in the first year of life, and is episodic.

2. In the adult, asthma begins at twenty to thirty years of age;

it tends to be continuous with episodic exacerbations; and it gets progressively worse with age.

3. The attacks in a child are seldom fatal because the spasm of the bronchi responds easily to bronchodilators.

4. The attacks in an adult are more dangerous than those in a child because the adult's terminal bronchioles become easily plugged with mucus and cellular debris and therefore do not respond well to the effect of nebulizers. On the other hand, a child may not use aerosols or nebulizers in the treatment of his asthma because these are addictive and may cause paradoxical bronchospasm and death.

5. In a child, emotional tension has far more importance in precipitating an attack than in an adult.

6. A respiratory distress in a child may look like asthma. It may be characterized by an effort to breathe, flaring of the nostrils, a quick heart beat, sweating, and wheezing sounds in the chest. Respiratory distress may be caused by an infection, spontaneous pneumothorax, or an accidental poisoning.

7. Asthma in a child should be handled more energetically than in an adult. We call this treatment "management," because it is not a cure, even though we may know what has caused the asthma attack, or how to control it.

8. With good "management," asthma in a child is seldom a fatal disease. However, the sense of suffocation during an attack, or the anticipation of more attacks, may damage the personality of the child and make him lose his self-confidence.

HISTORY OF ASTHMA

Asthma is an old disease that was known to the Chinese, Egyptians, Hebrews, Greeks, Romans, and Arabs. The earliest known treatise on asthma was written in Spain around the year 1150 by Moses Maimonides. This treatise remains up to the present day a masterpiece in the clinical study of the disease. A scientific cause-

and-effect study of asthma was done around the year 1870 by Salter, and then by Blackley. Salter reported a case of asthma caused by a cat, while Blackley proved its connection to pollen. Around 1900 Robert Koch, Von Pirquet, and Bela Shick connected the disease to allergy. This was followed by discoveries in skin testing for the causes of asthma, and desensitization for its treatment. However, the great and radical step in its history came about 1950, when steroids became known for their life-saving properties in intractable asthma.

IMMUNOLOGICAL ASTHMA

Definition and Diagnosis

The most common form of bronchial asthma is immunological or allergic asthma. However, many diseases have symptoms such as dyspnea, cyanosis, a chronic cough, and wheezing sounds in the chest exactly like immunological asthma. These diseases are caused by foreign bodies in the lungs, congenital malformations of vessels around the lungs, cysts and tumors in or around the lung, lymph glands enlarged by tuberculosis, and acute infections of the lung in children who suffer from immunological deficiencies. It is an illness that offers a spectrum of diagnostic pitfalls. A history of wheezing and coughing in an atopic child simplifies matters because it points toward classical immunological asthma. However, if a child has no personal or family history of allergy, the cause of his asthma is not easy to diagnose. The child may need a CBC, an X ray of the chest, a sweat test, a tuberculin test, a bronchoscopy, and immunological studies to clear up the diagnosis.

Causes

The causes of immunological asthma are allergens which may enter the body as inhalants in the air a child breathes, or as ingestants with his food or drink, or as contactants when it is something he touches or wears. Inhalant allergens are the pollen of trees, grasses, and weeds; the spores of molds; animal dander; and house dust. Food allergens are varied, and although any food is capable of sensitizing, there are some foods that are encountered with special frequency. These are milk, cereals, eggs, chocolate, nuts, shellfish, and fresh fruit. Injectant allergens that may cause asthma are penicillin, horse serum, bee and insect stings. Bacterial allergens, which may also cause asthma, are hard to implicate because we have no specific tests for them.

Symptoms

An acute attack of asthma begins with sneezing, a nasal discharge, a dry cough, some wheezing, some difficulty in breathing, and anxiety. As the attack progresses, the cough becomes productive and may be accompanied by vomiting, which relieves the chest of its mucus. Objectively, the chest is distended, and it has inspiratory rales which one can hear with a stethoscope or even at a distance. In between attacks, there may be no findings at all. Such an attack may follow an immediate exposure to an allergen (a food, animal dander, and so forth), a protracted exposure to an allergen (house dust constantly inhaled during a whole night of sleep), or a cumulative exposure to more than one allergen (an allergenic food eaten simultaneously with an exposure to dust or pollen).

Prevention

The preventive measures should be directed against:
1. Foods. Asthma due to foods is easily prevented by eliminating from the diet all those foods the child is sensitive to for a period of six months. Also, freezing, canning, or boiling make food less allergenic. At about four or five years of age, the child usually adapts himself to the foods to which he is sensitive, and he tolerates

them better. However, certain highly allergenic foods should never be reintroduced into his diet as a matter of principle. These foods are chocolate, nuts, all shellfish, and strawberries.

2. Inhalants. These should be avoided at all costs, as they are the most frequent cause of immunological asthma. A dust-free bedroom with an electrostatic air-purifier is a must. Also, vacations should be taken in a pollen-free area. Although there is a detailed description of these areas in the previous chapter (pages 106–116), the following will suffice for a quick glance: (a) Seattle, Washington; (b) California (entire state); (c) Grand Canyon National Park, Arizona; (d) Pike's Peak, Colorado; (e) Rocky Mountain National Park, Colorado; (f) Yellowstone National Park, Wyoming; (g) Isle Royale National Park, Michigan; (h) St. Francis, Maine; (i) Greenville Junction, Maine; (j) Blue Mountain Lake (Adirondacks), New York; (k) Bethlehem, New Hampshire; (l) Carroll, New Hampshire; (m) Suncrest (Catskills), New York; (n) Miami Beach, Florida; (o) Key West, Florida.

3. Pets. There should be none in the house of an asthmatic child.

4. Drugs. Unnecessary drugs (that is, drugs not prescribed by a doctor), such as aspirin, penicillin, laxatives, cold tablets, tranquilizers, sleeping pills, cough syrups, and skin ointments, among others, are not to be given to the asthmatic child at all. Injected drugs, such as penicillin, horse serum, and the venom of insects and bees (even though given by a doctor in desensitization) are to be avoided as much as possible.

5. Contactants. Although these—wool, leather, silk, nylon— rarely cause asthma, they are to be avoided as they may cause rashes that irritate the asthmatic child.

6. Colds. The common cold is to be avoided by the atopic child because he catches it easily and cannot get rid of it quickly. The child should avoid the members of his family who have colds, and wear a mask to avoid inhaling the bacteria that are sneezed into the air. He should be given antibiotics (erythromycin) if his cold lingers more than two days. A cold may cause bacterial asthma, and may open the door to inhalant asthma.

Bacteria as a Cause of Immunological Asthma

Bacterial allergy is a controversial subject, and there are arguments both for and against it. These arguments occur mainly in regard to the bacteria the tonsils harbor, their importance as a cause of asthma, and whether by removing the focus of infection through tonsillectomy we can cure or prevent an asthma caused by a bacterial infection.

The Asthmatic Child and Tonsillectomy

Removal of the tonsils of an allergenic child demands considerable thought. Tonsils may harbor bacteria, but at the same time they play a local role in providing immunity against infection. Each tonsillectomy has to be decided on individually. The operation, if carried out, has to be done in winter, when snow is on the ground, so that no undue exposure of the abraded tissue to dust, mold, and pollen takes place. Even though there is no general agreement on the role that bacteria play in asthma, there is a general agreement on the fact that a relationship between frequent tonsillar infections and asthma does exist, and that some nonspecific factors that in themselves do *not* cause asthma may cause it, provided an initial asthma attack was brought about by an infection in the tonsils. These nonspecific factors are climate variation, chemical irritants, sudden chilling, excessive sweating, inhalation of fumes, and emotional upheaval. The question then arises as to whether we should remove the tonsils of all atopic children to steer them away from the bacteria found in their tonsils, or avoid this procedure because it is potentially dangerous. There are three possible answers to this question: (1) yes—removal of the tonsils takes away the bacteria which are the cause of infection and asthma; (2) no—removal of the tonsils prevents the formation of adequate local immunity against these bacteria, and therefore causes more asthma in the long run; (3) it all depends on the individual evaluation of the case.

The indications for tonsillectomy in the atopic and the nonatopic child are the same. They depend on the presence of a chronic infection in the tonsils that no antibiotic has been able to reach, as well as on the frequency and severity of the infections in the tonsils.

NONSPECIFIC CAUSES OF ASTHMA: PERIODIC ASTHMA

Some chemical irritants—paints, varnishes, lacquer, turpentine, insecticides, tobacco smoke, perfumes, food odors, or gasoline odor —may be able to upset the allergic balance and precipitate an asthma attack. Also, quick changes in temperature and humidity, plus other numerous environmental changes still unaccounted for, may also cause wheezing. A specific example of wheezing caused by loosely defined environmental factors follows.

It is common knowledge in Israel, northern Spain, Italy, New Zealand, and Argentina that asthmatic children become irritable, surly, and on edge during some months of the year. The number and severity of their attacks increases sharply, and they become so sensitive that they can even predict an attack a day in advance.

What causes this? In Israel abrupt changes in barometric pressure, temperature, and wind velocity occur during Khamsin, which is a period of fifty days that occur from May to July. During these fifty days, a special wind blows from the desert into the Tel Aviv area, and Israeli scientists believe that this wind causes a change in the electrical charge of the atmosphere from the good negative ions to the bad positive ones. It is this change alone, and not the barometric oscillations or humidity variations, that the Israeli scientists believe is the cause of the increase in the frequency of asthma attacks during this period of the year. This belief has led a private company in Israel to manufacture a special machine called Ionotron, which enriches the air with healthful negative ions. This device recirculates the air at home several times each hour, each time changing the positively charged ions into negatively charged ions, thus giving mountain-fresh air right to the home of the allergic child. The device is easy to carry, plugs in any 110 V outlets, and has no hazardous emission of ozone.

This subject was studied some years ago by the American Society of Heating, Refrigeration, and Air-Conditioning. They concluded that the good effect of ionization on asthma was due to unrecorded variables in humidity, temperature changes, barometric pressure changes, airborne contaminants, and the psychological disposition of the asthmatic child. They also found out that air-cleaners that work by precipitating impurities through ionization have no effect on the ion level of the conditioned space. The author has no personal experience with ionization in the treatment of allergies, but those who believe in ionization should be aware that the electronic air-cleaning device as well as the ionizing machine have to be installed together in the bedroom of the atopic child.

In New York, Dr. Vincent J. Fontana has done experimental work on atmospheric variation as a cause of asthma. He has demonstrated that abrupt changes in humidity and temperature do not cause asthma or increase its frequency, intensity, or recurrence. However, should these atmospheric variations add their weight to air pollution or airborne inhalant allergens already present in the atmosphere, they may cause an intensification or complication in the regular course of the disease. Therefore, moving an asthmatic child from, let us say, New York to Arizona or California to avoid the above-mentioned abrupt atmospheric changes cannot be useful unless the area to which the child moves is free of inhalant allergens.

We may conclude that immunological asthma is usually brought about by a hereditary predisposition plus an exposure to allergens. However, once it is established as a disease, atmospheric variations conducive to change in electrical ionization can trigger it off easily and periodically.

DIFFERENTIAL DIAGNOSIS BETWEEN
IMMUNOLOGICAL AND NONSPECIFIC ASTHMA

Immunological asthma does not occur as an isolated incident in the life of an atopic child, but rather as one of the manifestations of an atopic constitution. These manifestations are nasal secretions; a dry, itchy, scaly skin with flare-ups of eczema; urticaria (hives) present at intervals; migraine headaches; tension fatigue; diarrhea; abdominal pains; geographical tongue; bloating or canker sores; and so forth. Nonimmunological asthma, or simply a wheezing sound in the chest, usually gives other clues to its origin. A foreign body in the lungs gives only local wheezing; an infection responds to antibiotics; emphysema is made worse with exertion; a congenital heart disease is accompanied by cyanosis; and so forth. Furthermore, immunological asthma responds readily to two drugs: adrenalin and aminophylline.

CONTROL OF AN ACUTE ATTACK BY A PARENT

No parent should diagnose or treat any allergic condition; this must be left to the family physician. There is, however, one exception to this rule. Acute asthma attacks must be handled by parents, otherwise life-threatening situations might arise because of precious time lost while waiting for a doctor. Furthermore, the fear and sense of helplessness brought about by an asthmatic attack can be appreciably lightened if the child and his family have some authoritative knowledge on how to give immediate relief so that the child gains self-confidence and does not fear suffocation.

Some general measures are helpful in any type of asthma. As soon as an asthma attack begins, the parents should put the child into a dust-free, animal-free bedroom and then evaluate the seriousness of the situation. If they are dealing with a light wheeze with no difficulty in breathing, an antihistaminic cough syrup might do.

A syrup such as Chlor-trimeton Expectorant or Dimetane Expectorant, plain or DC, must be kept in the medicine cabinet. (DC pertains to the codeine content of the syrup, and the DC syrup should be used if the child is anxious or fearful.) If fifteen minutes pass and the parents notice a worsening of the condition, the child should be given a teaspoon of Tedral Syrup or Marax. If another fifteen minutes pass and the parents see no improvement, the child should be given an injection (⅓ cc.) of adrenalin. If one hour passes and the adrenalin fails to work, an aminophylline enema should be given. If this also fails to give relief, a doctor must be called.

Any asthma attack that lasts two days or more probably needs an antibiotic, especially if the mucus has become thick, yellow, or green. A bottle of erythromycin should be kept in the medicine cabinet for such a situation. Penicillin should never be used.

If the child is constipated, an enema will liberate him from the feces and gases that press on his chest and thus make his breathing more difficult.

All during the attack, the parents should try to keep a relaxed frame of mind. A note of interest—though of doubtful aid—to the parent treating an acute asthma attack: certain situations may unexpectedly relieve the attack. Among these are a high fever, almost any kind of major surgery, unbearable pain, and extreme mental stress. The factors involved in such a natural relief of asthma will not be discussed here, but it is important to know that such relief is possible and may come when it is least expected.

SPECIFIC AND SYMPTOMATIC TREATMENT OF CHRONIC ASTHMA

Frequent asthmatic attacks, even though relieved with medication, constitute chronic asthma. The "management" of chronic asthma consists in identifying its precipitating factors, diminishing the exposure to these factors, hyposensitization against them, and using symptomatic medication. The latter is made up of bronchodilators, mucolytics, and corticosteroids.

Identifying the precipitating factors may require skin testing. Skin testing is the easiest means for identifying implicated inhalant allergens. It is not, however, helpful in diagnosing asthma caused by foods or bacteria.

Diminishing the sensitivity to the precipitating factors requires desensitization. Desensitization usually gives satisfactory results unless some outside factors prevent it from doing so. Some of these factors are a family that does not cooperate by bringing the child in regularly for his injections; lack of avoidance of the allergens injected; new sensitivities that may develop after the desensitization treatment has started; a new and unexpected psychic stress (the death of a parent, the birth of a sibling); incomplete elimination of allergenic foods; the presence of pets in the household; and so forth.

Even though symptomatic medication of acute asthma has already been discussed in this chapter, a word about a new therapeutic modality deserves special mention. This consists of inhalations of a new drug called *cromolyn sodium,* a symptomatic and nonspecific agent unrelated to any drug used in the treatment of asthma. It is capable of "inhibiting" the episodes of inhalant asthma, and it does not possess any toxicity to the kidneys, liver, or blood. It is given orally through a turbo-inhaler device four times daily. If taken for a long period of time, it improves the child's capacity to play and exercise, reduces his school absenteeism, his hospitalizations, and his use of other symptomatic medication. Its trial is justified when there is an unavoidable exposure to inhalant allergens during high pollen-count days, and in chronic asthma with multiple etiology that does not respond to standard treatment.

If the child does not respond to specific and symptomatic medication, his condition is called *status asthmaticus.* This is a very serious illness that should not exist if proper out-patient management has been given to the child. It endangers life and requires hospitalization. (See the following chapter for a fuller discussion.) If the child survives his status asthmaticus but continues to have daily difficulty with asthma, even though on a small scale, he has intractable asthma.

8 Intractable Asthma and Its Rehabilitation

Intractable or "unmanageable" asthma is a constant difficulty in breathing accompanied by a wheeze. It may be brought about by frequent asthma attacks at short intervals, excessive use of cough suppressants, or insufficient fluid intake while having asthma. These conditions prevent easy expectoration and cause an accumulation of dry and thick mucus, which clogs the bronchi. This clogging makes asthma a disease which is hard to "manage" because adrenalin or aminophyllin, which give relief in asthma by relaxing the muscles of the bronchi, have no effect on softening the mucus that resides in them.

A child with intractable asthma usually ends up becoming easy prey to cortisone abuse, and his further treatment will have to be done in a hospital. Hospitalization, however, is a traumatizing experience, and its effects on the mental health of the child should be weighed carefully before it is recommended.

THE EMOTIONAL ASPECTS OF HOSPITALIZATION IN ASTHMA

Asthma is an emotionally frightening experience; hospitalization makes it more difficult to accept because of separation from home and parents, impersonal care, lonely surroundings, and fear of death. An asthmatic child should be hospitalized only when absolutely necessary. While in the hospital, he must be allowed to wear his usual clothing; his room must be made homelike, with gay decorations, some toys, his favorite possessions, books, and soft music; his nurse should wear pastel-colored uniforms and provide him with games appropriate to his age and mentality. As soon as is feasible, he should be allowed to leave his bed, eat in the children's cafeteria, and associate with his mates. His physician must create an open, permissive atmosphere in which the child is free to ask questions and receive clear, plausible explanations about the nature and severity of his asthma. However, this is not tantamount to frank discussion on the possible dangers of the disease and its related medical problems. All in all, the hospital should simulate home as much as possible and emotional trauma should be avoided during the child's stay there.

Hospitalization may succeed in keeping a child free of asthma. He may remain a well-compensated chronic asthmatic for many years unless his precarious balance is upset by (1) a new upper respiratory infection; (2) continuous exposure to the allergen that has caused his chronic asthma (presence of a dog in the house); (3) continued exposure to some nonspecific irritants, such as tobacco and air pollution (living in a big city); (4) an emotional upset (death of a mother); (5) medication abuse (steroids, nebulizations of Iso); (6) dehydration (sweating and lack of fluid intake); (7) fatigue brought about by a constant struggle to breathe.

If the child's allergic balance is upset by one of the above-mentioned factors, he may experience more spasms in his bronchi. In this case, adrenalin and aminophylline do not give relief because the bronchi have already become mechanically clogged with thick, infected, and dry mucus. The child cannot breathe properly and goes into a status asthmaticus, that is, he becomes cyanotic, apprehensive, and agitated; he leans forward in his bed, sweats, and strains to expand his chest; he has a quick heart beat and a wheezing sound in the lungs that one can hear at a distance; his chest becomes hyperresonant, and his breath sounds are diminished. He needs active and courageous treatment by a specialist; otherwise death may follow. This is asthma at its worst, and its treatment consists of (1) hydration, by means of intravenous fluids (five to six liters daily); (2) nebulization through a cold-mist vaporizer; (3) aeration, by pushing oxygen into the lungs with an intermittent positive-pressure machine, or by endotracheal intubation, or with a tracheotomy, or by direct administration with a cannula or a mask; (4) bronchodilation through adrenalin, Iso, aminophylline, or steriods; (5) sedation by means of Thorazine, chloral hydrate, or Atarax; (6) other useful procedures, such as injection of antibiotics (stagnating mucus always gets infected), and establishment of an electrolyte balance.

A SUMMARY OF THE TOTAL "MANAGEMENT" OF ASTHMA IN A CHILD

Asthma begets asthma. Its best treatment is not to have it. A child can achieve this by avoiding birth into an atopic family—although this, of course, is hardly up to the child—as well as not being exposed after birth to allergens and air pollutants. Acute asthmatics do very well with adrenalin, while mild, moderate, or chronic asthmatics do better with ephedrine and aminophylline every six hours around the clock. Asthma caused by infection needs antibiotics, and the antibotic of choice is erythromycin, not penicillin. To lower the temperature in infections, Tylenol is to be used, not aspirin.

In general, an asthmatic child should seek to have soft mucus, which is easy to expectorate. This can be achieved by giving him lots of fluids to drink, plus iodides and glyceryl guaiacolate by mouth to break up the mucus. If he is unable to expectorate because his mucus is deeply lodged in a bronchiectatic cavity, or because his lungs are emphysematous, the use of postural drainage exercises and bronchodilator aerosols help. Steroids should be reserved for cases where nothing else is expected to work.

Adequate rest, normal athletic activities, breathing exercises, psychotherapy, and avoidance of stress are all supplementary but essential parts in the treatment of chronic asthma. Its basic treatment is, however, hyposensitization. This lessens the impact, lengthens the time span between one attack and another, and at times may make the child completely healthy.

A chronic asthmatic child may have to be relocated either permanently or temporarily in a specialized institute if he gets intractable asthma.

REHABILITATION OF INTRACTABLE ASTHMA

The purpose of rehabilitation is not only to add years to the life of a chronically ill child, but also to add life to his years. This is done with breathing exercises and psychiatry.

The American Academy of Pediatrics advises the following breathing exercises for physical rehabilitation.

Preface to Parents

The asthmatic child tends to develop faulty breathing habits; he loses the mobility of his lower chest and his upper chest becomes overworked. He needs to learn to increase the movement of his lower chest. The abdominal muscles must be trained to assist the diaphragm in some of the work of breathing, enabling the asthmatic child to breathe more easily and efficiently.

The improvement in respiratory function demonstrated in normal children after exercise has encouraged pediatric allergists to add breathing exercises to the total treatment program for asthmatic children. The goals sought are to teach the child:

1. To learn the basic breathing exercises for the maximum use of respiratory muscles, especially the diaphragmatic muscle.

2. To learn to use these exercises to stop an asthmatic episode early.

3. To improve exercise tolerance and correct postural defects.

4. To develop self-confidence.

These breathing exercises will have to be taught to the child initially by the physician or therapist. Designed to help children institute and maintain correct breathing patterns, the exercises are most beneficial when performed daily, preferably on arising and before bedtime.

It should be emphasized that these breathing exercises are not curative. They do, however, represent an additional aid in the entire management program needed to prevent recurrence of asthma in children.

The Exercises

Do you know how to breathe? Sure you do . . . but do you know there is a *right* way and a *wrong* way to breathe?

Let me show you how you can learn the *right* way to breathe.

First, let's look inside your chest to see how we breathe.

The way you start is:

1. Lie down on the floor.
2. Bend your knees and keep your feet on the floor.
3. Put your arms at your sides.

Now . . . take a *deep* breath . . . and let it out . . . slowly. See what moves? Your chest and abdomen go up and down. Do it again . . . a few times.

Now try this. Put one hand on the top part of your chest . . . put your other hand on your abdomen . . . and breathe in through your nose.

Your *abdomen* should go *out* like a balloon. Your chest should not move.

Inhaling is using the *diaphragm.*

Try it again . . . as you pull air in through the *nose,* the hand on your chest is still . . . only the hand on your abdomen goes *up.* As you blow the air *out* through *pursed lips,* the hand on your abdomen goes *down* . . . the hand on your chest stays still.

Now let's practice *abdominal breathing:* Fold your hands on your abdomen like this . . . now breathe in through your nose . . . see your abdomen get round like a ball? Do this ten times, making sure your chest remains still.

Now let's try the *most important* part of breathing, exhaling. Blow *all* the air out through your mouth, using pursed lips. Use the hand on your abdomen to help *press* all the air out.

Now your abdomen should be flat. Do this ten times, *slowly.*

Just for fun, put a *book* on your abdomen. See if you can make the book *fall off* as you take in air and make your abdomen round. Your abdomen should get *flat* again as you blow all the air out.

Remember to keep your chest still.

Here is another way:

Sit in a chair, nice and tall. Hold a book against your abdomen. Breathe in some air and let your abdomen *push out* against the book. Now, *push the book* hard against your abdomen.

Bend over . . . at the time *blowing out* air. Do it the same way, ten times, *slowly.*

Try this the next time . . . and every time . . . you feel short of breath: Sit leaning forward with a straight back, the arms resting on the knees. Now, breathe in through the nose, then blow *all* the air out through the mouth slowly, keeping your chest still. Breathing this way will make you feel better and less tired.

If the exercises make you *cough,* this is good—it will help to dislodge any sputum.

Try lying over the side of the bed for ten to fifteen minutes to *drain out* the sputum. Mother can help you cough it out by clapping gently on your back. You will feel much better every time you do this!

Can you walk with a book balanced on your head? You can keep a *good posture* by remembering to stand up straight with your shoulders relaxed. Don't forget to keep your back flat against the chair when sitting.

Now you know how to breathe. See if you can do it this way *all the time.*

> *sitting*
> *standing*
> *running*
> *playing*
> *working*

at home . . . at school . . . everywhere.

Let's keep a record . . . Make an *X* each day you do your breathing exercises.

Sunday

Monday

Tuesday

Wednesday

Thursday

Friday

Saturday

Another approach to the same principle in breathing is provided by Breon Laboratories of New York. We state them here for variety, and also because they are designed for home use by the child after he returns from an institute.

Breathing Exercises for Home Use

These exercises are designed to train your abdominal muscles to assist your diaphragm in some of the work of breathing. As you become accustomed to this different kind of breathing, you can expect to feel better and be more active in daily life.

Preparation

Breathing exercises are usually performed two to four times daily: on arising, before meals, during the late afternoon, or just before retiring. Each exercise period should last from one-half hour to one hour, depending on your physician's directions.

Before beginning your exercises, remove tight or restrictive clothing. Be sure your nasal passages are clear. If prescribed by your physician, inhale an aerosol medication according to his directions. This will relax and open the airways in your lungs, and will loosen tenacious mucus so it can be more easily expectorated.

Most important, do not hurry your breathing exercises. Rest when necessary. Do each as long as instructed. And in all cases, begin your day with the Basic Morning Exercise.

Basic Morning Exercise

Sit erect on the edge of a bed or chair and place hands over lower ribs and upper abdomen. Keep shoulders down, elbows straight out, fingers rigid. Repeat exercise ten times, or as physician directs.

Exhale while applying firm pressure against ribs and abdomen with hands. Exhale slowly through pursed lips—lips held partly open as when you are about to whistle.

Inhale after releasing pressure of hands slightly, but still applying effort against chest and abdomen. Cough gently to raise mucus.

Exercise One

Lie flat on the floor (not on a bed) and rest left hand across chest, right hand on abdomen. Inhale deeply through nose, letting abdomen rise. Then breathe out through pursed lips, pressing inward and upward firmly on abdomen. Try to move the chest as little as possible, letting the abdomen move up and down as you inhale and exhale. As your physician directs, you may practice this exercise while sitting or standing. Repeat six to eight times. Once you have developed this technique you should breathe in this manner even while walking.

Exercise Two

Lie flat on the floor and rest left hand across chest, right hand on abdomen. Bend knees, keeping them together. Keep feet on floor, bringing thighs toward chest as far as possible. Inhale through nose, letting abdomen rise. Then breathe out through pursed lips, pressing inward and upward firmly on abdomen. Repeat six to eight times, or as physician directs.

Exercise Three

Lie flat on the floor, raise knees, and lock arms around legs. Inhale through nose, letting abdomen rise. Lift feet from floor and exhale through pursed lips, pulling legs toward chest as far as possible with arms. Repeat six to eight times, or as physician directs.

Exercise Four

With feet elevated about fourteen inches and body in a straight line, rest left hand across chest, right hand on abdomen. Inhale deeply through nose, letting abdomen rise. Then breathe out through pursed lips, pressing inward and upward firmly on the abdomen. Try to move the chest as little as possible, letting the abdomen move up and down as you inhale and exhale. Repeat six to eight times, or as physician directs.

EMOTIONAL REHABILITATION OF A
CHRONICALLY ILL ASTHMATIC CHILD

To grasp what this rehabilitation implies, we must understand the role that emotions play in the life of an asthmatic child at home and in school.

At home, the life of such a child is an endless struggle to resolve the basic needs of living. It's the constant supervision of the parents, frequent sickness, and the off-and-on use of medication. The struggle gets worse as the family routine becomes disrupted by the child's special foods, his special clothing, the special heating and humidification of the house, the avoidance of pets, and the extra expense incurred through doctor's fees and medicines. This sort of life inevitably leads to sibling rivalry and rejection by parents.

In school, the life of an asthmatic child involves constant trouble because of poor performance. Consequently, his schoolmates and his teachers get nervous and angry with him and criticize him constantly. Such criticism causes emotional and behavioral reactions, which in turn bring more criticism. If such a child becomes aware of his emotional involvement, he adopts a defensive attitude. He becomes sullen, disagreeable, hostile and stubborn. He underachieves, cuts school, and fails.

The vicious cycle of events at home and in school can be summarized then as follows: a food or an inhalant allergen may cause abdominal pain, a sinus congestion, asthma, or plain nervous tension. The child does not feel well; he has a hard time at home and in school. Criticism brings failure, more criticism, tension, anxiety, and depression. The child no longer cares about avoiding allergens, becomes physically sick, and cuts school altogether. Consequently, he fails in it and avoids it still more.

The response of the asthmatic child to the above-mentioned threats depends on his moral fiber and character. Unfortunately, not all parents are capable of tackling the complicated job of giving a firm basis to a constantly threatened existence. Where parenthood has failed to supply the extra needed compassion, love, and understanding to each child who demands more than his share, an "engulfment" follows in which the parents live in guilt, and the rejected child lives in fear and anxiety.

No matter how confused the upbringing is, or how deep the "engulfment" of the child with his parents, resentfulness, anxiety, or depression may result—but not allergies. Allergies are brought about by a hereditary predisposition, frequent upper respiratory infections, and exposure to allergens. Furthermore, they do not usually cause an undue scarring of a child's personality. However, if a child happens to have a combination of wrong heredity and wrong upbringing, we have an allergy-prone child who is burdened with emotional problems. The life of such a child would then depend on how badly both of these factors interact.

In case the emotional factor is more important than the allergic one, it may superimpose itself on the regular pattern of the allergic factor, blur its contours, and make itself the main cause of the illness. Emotion all by itself may then bring about asthma attacks, and no exposure to an allergen would be necessary; the attacks emotion would bring about would be as dangerous as the ones caused by allergy. Let us not forget that the asthmatic child is a child above all. He has the anxieties, frustrations, and fears that pertain to all children of his age. Added to these he has the extra emotional burdens that his crippling disease puts on his budding personality.

The parents of such a child have to be observant, sensitive, and understanding of these emotional needs. It is their thoughts, reactions, and feelings that determine how bad the child's fears become and how his behavior will be. This behavior will make him self-confident or timid. If he is self-confident he may be sick, but not a mental cripple, and emotionally secure, even though asthmatic. If he is secure, he will be able to achieve in school, hobbies, or work, and be a worthy member of society. His greatest hurdle, however, is caused by stress during his school years. How he resolves his difficulties there determines the trend of his future life.

The following abbreviated case histories illustrate these points.

Case 1

Joan is a well-adjusted asthmatic child who wants no sympathy or attention. She achieves well in school and is loved by her teacher, her friends, and her parents. How did she achieve this good emotional adjustment and how has she learned to live with the physical limitations of her asthma?

Joan's parents were loving but not overprotective. They have always included her in all family and school activities, while still paying attention to her condition. Joan saw herself developing certain unexplained talents and making friends. She is secure in her world.

Joan, despite her handicap, is in every respect like all other children. She realizes that it is only human to want to be protected and have others be compassionate to her. She knows, however, that this will cripple her personality and make her a dependent with no incentive at all. She takes a realistic attitude toward her condition because she knows that she will always be asthmatic. She asks for no extra attention and does not need any.

Case 2

John is a chronic asthmatic who attends school, even though he is intermittently under asthma medication. In general he is indifferent about his schoolwork, and is socially withdrawn because he is small in size and therefore a subject of ridicule to his friends. His parents do not get along and they quarrel frequently. Both of them work, get tired toward the evening, and rush to give John his medication even though he wheezes only slightly. John keeps getting worse every day and demands more medication. How can such a child be helped?

We have to determine why John's asthma is worse. A conference with the parents, the school psychologist, and the school doctor brought out the following fact: John is allergic to certain foods. His mother does not prepare his lunch, but lets him eat freely in the school cafeteria, where these same foods are served. When he eats those foods, he gets asthma, and is then unable to follow his schoolwork. He fails, and gets depressed. Getting home, he wishes he could discuss his problems with his parents, but they have no time for him. He brings about an asthma attack in order to get their attention. They respond with symptomatic medication and more rejection.

The treatment advised by the school doctor consisted of cutting the vicious cycle by putting John in an institution for a while and letting the parents at the same time get some counseling by the school psychologist. Two months later the mother brought John back home, and stopped working. She prepared his lunch at home, and devoted more time to her sick son. John's attacks decreased and his morale became higher. He got along better with his teacher and his classmates and his grades in school became passable. John's personality was salvaged because the school doctor and the school psychologist both had a real interest in uncovering the causes of the psychological and organic factors that sustained his asthma.

Case 3

Thomas is six years old, has had asthma since birth, and is taking steroids on the advice of his doctor. He finds difficulty in expressing his feelings and resorts instead to nail biting and stuttering. His parents and schoolmates ridicule him about these "mannerisms." This makes him angry and brings about frequent attacks of asthma.

Thomas lives in Manhattan, where he is further victimized by the polluted air. He gets frequent upper respiratory infections, which stop him from going to school. He has been left back because of underachievement.

As compared to the two instances mentioned above in which the course of asthma was reversed, Thomas was not lucky enough to have the proper medication or guidance. His case ended sadly by his developing emphysema in addition to his asthma. He is now at a point of no return, because there is no cure for emphysema.

Asthmatic children respond to stress with more asthma. School represents a stress and therefore a cause of more asthma because it forces the child to live in a group, and to achieve. The parent of an asthmatic child must set realistic goals for the child in his studies, sports, and social contacts.

The treatment of asthma when complicated by emotions has to

follow two distinct paths. The asthmatic child has to be treated as a whole, and not merely as an asthmatic. The scars on his personality have to be treated, as well as the wounds of his body. If the scars on his personality are too deep, he may need a special institute, one of those to be mentioned later, where allergic treatment goes along with parentectomy, that is, the division of the child from his parents for a prolonged period of time, a time needed for child and parent to be treated and rehabilitated.

The healthy emotional balance between parent and child is well described in *The Prophet* by Kahlil Gibran who was born in Lebanon and raised in America. He died in 1931 in St. Vincent's Hospital of New York, where I now work. His views on the subject are classical reading in psychology and philosophy in all major colleges.

> Your children are not your children.
> They are the sons and daughters of Life's longing for itself.
> They come through you but not from you,
> And though they are with you yet they belong not to you.

> You may give them your love but not your thoughts,
> For they have their own thoughts.
> You may house their bodies but not their souls,
> For their souls dwell in the house of tomorrow, which you cannot visit, not even in your dreams.
> You may strive to be like them, but seek not to make them like you.
> For life goes not backward nor tarries with yesterday.

> You are the bows from which your children as living arrows are sent forth.
> The archer sees the mark upon the path of the infinite, and He bends you with His might that His arrows may go swift and far.

Let your bending in the archer's hand be for gladness;
For even as He loves the arrow that flies, so He loves
also the bow that is stable.

Kahlil Gibran

CHOOSING A PERMANENT RELOCATION AREA FOR THE CHRONIC ASTHMATIC

A child who suffers from intractable asthma that is progressing toward emphysema needs a permanent relocation. Before recommending the move, we have to weigh the psychic, social, and economic problems that the intended move will create. We have to keep in mind that no place in the world can free a child of allergies, because it is in his nature to develop new sensitivities. However, if for various reasons we have come to the conclusion that the child must absolutely relocate, we have to study the allergies of the child, as well as the inhalants present in the air of the new area.

The new area would have to be chosen in light of the following facts:

1. An atopic child who suffers from infections because of air pollution needs a dry climate with minimal air pollution. Any place in the Southwest, especially if it is situated at an altitude of one to two thousand feet and far away from any industrial zone, will do.

2. A child with sensitivity to pollen, such as ragweed, will improve in any location west of the Rockies. Also, most of Canada and Europe are safe areas for sufferers from ragweed because ragweed does not grow there. On the other hand, if the child is sensitive to grasses, he will do better in any eastern city that has a short grass-pollinating season. Some areas, such as California and Israel, are especially dangerous for sufferers from grass pollen, because grasses pollinate there during eight months of the year.

3. A child coming from the subtropics and suffering from allergy to insect dust can relocate anywhere in the North.

4. Mold allergy is especially bad in the temperate regions of coastal areas. The temperate coastal areas of Israel, Cuba, and

many Latin American countries are especially noted for their high air-mold content. In general, any mountain resort above six thousand feet is a fairly safe place for a mold-sensitive child.

5. The special geography of the relocation area is most important: (*a*) mountain air has a reduced partial oxygen pressure, so a prolonged stay in the mountains may cause improved lung ventilation, increased peripheral blood circulation, increased hemoglobin concentration, and adrenal gland stimulation; (*b*) forests have an air that has little biological cooling, a high humidity, a reduced solar radiation, longer-lasting fogs, and less electrostatic variations —characteristics that are unhealthy to the chronic asthmatic child; (*c*) sea air has great turbulence, a strong cooling effect, great intensity of solar radiation, little temperature variation, high humidity, and a small amount of dust, pollen, chemicals, or pollutants— air qualities that are healthy for a chronically ill asthmatic child.

In conclusion, although there is no safe place to relocate a chronically ill asthmatic child, some geographical areas may be better suited for his purposes than others. Relocation would depend on the type of inhalant allergens causing the asthma, as well as on the special geography of the chosen locality.

A Case History: Geography and Asthma

Subject: P.J. (male)

Age: 10 years

Symptoms: P.J. has suffered from these multiple inhalant allergies during the past five years: dust, molds, and ragweed.

During Christmas vacation he goes skiing and his allergies disappear. When he returns to his apartment in Manhattan, they come back. During the summer he goes to his uncle's cottage in Long Beach, where he wheezes on and off all during the summer months. In August, the wheezing gets worse.

P.J.'s allergies are organic and environmental. The high mountains are free of molds and ragweed, while his uncle's cottage is damp, moldy, and has ragweed in its vicinity. Conclusions:

1. P.J. does not feel well in Manhattan because the air is polluted there. This brings about frequent lung infections, which opens the door to

the inhalation of dust in his apartment, and predisposes him to bacterial allergy.

2. P.J. feels well in high mountains that are covered with snow because they have no molds (mold's mother dwelling is covered with snow), and no ragweed grows there. Also, mountain air improves lung ventilation and peripheral circulation, increases hemoglobin concentration and stimulates the adrenal glands.

3. P.J. gets asthma in his uncle's cottage in Long Beach because of its location near the sea and the presence of ragweed in its back yard. The sea as well as plants bring about humidity and fog in the air, and encourage further growth of ragweed and molds.

On pages 152–157 is a listing of institutes in the United States and Canada that specialize in the rehabilitation of chronic asthma through temporary relocation, psychotherapy, and breathing exercises.

A Case History: Indiscriminate Use of Corticosteroids in Intractable Asthma and Emphysema

Subject: J.B.

Age: 11 years

Symptoms: J.B. came to New York from Tel Aviv, where he had suffered from asthma for eight years and where he was treated with corticosteroids daily. His relocation came about in January, when snow was on the ground. J.B.'s asthma disappeared overnight. A pediatrician's examination revealed a stuffy nose, fluid in the middle ear, eczema on the outer ear, rales in the chest but no wheezing. Skin testing showed strong positive reactions to molds and dust.

Treatment: No desensitization treatment was advised at the time. Potassium iodide drops were prescribed by mouth, along with an electrostatic air-filter for his bedroom. Corticosteroids were allowed on and off to ward off bad asthmatic attacks. Four years later, August to November, J.B. developed sneezing bouts, a runny nose, itching, a general malaise, slight temperature elevation, and wheezing. For two subsequent fall seasons, J.B.'s symptoms recurred. The third fall, J.B.'s father took him to Germany, where he found some relief. The next year, returning to America, he became very ill again.

Comments: J.B.'s asthma exacerbation was caused by sensitivity to rag-weed pollen, which appeared over and above the original asthma he suffered in Tel Aviv, which was caused by molds. This time J.B. was again skin tested, found to be sensitive to ragweed in addition to molds, and put on perennial desensitization injections of ragweed pollen. Even though his steroid medication was in-creased, J.B.'s wheezing did not abate during the fall. He had constant difficulty breathing, and with the least effort he needed oxygen. His color was cyanotic and his mucus thick. X rays re-vealed emphysema in his lungs. J.B.'s allergist advised a rehabilita-tion center in Denver, Colorado, so that J.B. could get physical therapy in the form of breathing exercises and psychotherapy in order to relieve his depressions. J.B. was unable to go to Denver, but moved to rural Vermont. His asthma was controlled to some extent there, but not his emphysema. Oxygen and antibiotics were prescribed on and off, and drops of potassium iodide were given regularly to soften his mucus. His life expectancy was sharply reduced because of frequent lung infections.

Notes: (1) At the beginning of his illness, J.B. was neither properly tested nor properly desensitized. (2) J.B. was treated indiscrimi-nately with corticosteroids, to which he became addicted. His gen-eral powers of reaction and his resistance to allergens and stress were thus diminished. He became susceptible to frequent infec-tions. (3) Living in New York was detrimental to J.B.'s health because of (a) air pollution; (b) the presence of ragweed pollen in the air of New York; (c) the quick pace of life.

Conclusion: Indiscriminate use of corticosteroids in the treatment of asthma without a proper history, skin testing, desensitization, and avoidance of allergens, is dangerous. The result may be intractable asthma, bronchiectasis, emphysema, and possibly death.

THE USE OF HYPNOSIS IN CHRONIC ASTHMA

A lot has been written about the use of hypnosis in the treatment of chronic asthma. The author has had a one-year experience in the subject, and cites this case history to summarize his views on the value of such a treatment.

A fourteen-year-old boy, who knew that his lifelong asthma was caused by allergy to egg, was brought to my office to have this ailment treated with hypnosis. His father and mother insisted that his condition was caused by nerves and not by allergy, even though an intracutaneous test confirmed his allergy to egg.

Under hypnosis, the boy was made to drink one drop of boiled egg yolk in a glass of water, and nothing happened. When this was followed by one drop of boiled egg white, a slight wheeze developed. Another drop of fresh egg white provoked a full-blown asthma attack that had to be stopped with an adrenalin injection.

The conclusion is that allergic asthma is not to be treated with hypnosis, even though its psychological component may be improved through its use. For this purpose, the use of tranquilizers is cheaper and safer.

Institutes for the Rehabilitation of Chronic Asthma

ADDRESS	NAME OF INSTITUTE	MEDICAL DIRECTOR
CALIFORNIA		
Palo Alto (94304) 520 Willow Road	Stanford Children's Convalescent Hospital	M. Harry Jennison, M.D.
Tujunga (91042) 775 McGroarty Avenue	Sunair Home for Asthmatic Children	Lawrence Strick, M.D.
COLORADO		
Denver (80206) 3800 East Colfax Avenue	National Jewish Hospital	Elliot F. Ellis, M.D.
Denver (80204) 3401 West 19th Avenue	Children's Asthma Research Institute and Hospital	E. Middleton, Jr., M.D. C. J. Falliers, M.D.
DISTRICT OF COLUMBIA		
Washington (20017) 1731 Bunker Hill Road NE	Hospital for Sick Children	Robert Snell, M.D.
FLORIDA		
North Miami Beach (33162) 1800 Northeast 168th Street	Asthmatic Children's Foundation Residential Treatment Center	Meyer B. Marks, M.D.
ILLINOIS		
Chicago (60649) 65th at Lake Michigan	LaRabida Children's Hospital Research Center	Burton J. Grossman, M.D.

AREA SERVED		BED CAPACITY		AGE		LENGTH OF STAY		
	Out of							
ocal	State	Total	Asthma	Min.	Max.	Min.	Avg.	Max.
es	Western	65	as needed		18			
es	South-western	39	39	5	12	2 mos.	12 mos.	24 mos.
es	Yes	120	75				7 mos.	
es (0%)	Yes (90%)	165	165	6	16	2 wks.	12–18 mos.	36 mos.
es	No	75	25		16	3 mos.	6 mos.	
es	Yes	36	36	5	13	3 mos.	18 mos.	2 yrs.
Yes	Yes	104	as needed		20			

Institutes for the Rehabilitation of Chronic Asthma (continued)

ADDRESS	NAME OF INSTITUTE	MEDICAL DIRECTOR
KENTUCKY		
Lexington (40504) 2050 Versailles Road	Cardinal Hill Convalescent Hospital	Kenneth L. Gerson, M.D.
MARYLAND		
Baltimore (21209) 1708 West Rogers Avenue	Happy Hills Hospital Incorporated	Eugene Caplan, M.D.
MASSACHUSETTS		
Lakeville (02346)	Lakeville Hospital Asthma Rehabilitation Unit	Irving Bailit, M.D.
MICHIGAN		
Grand Rapids (49506) 920 Cherry Street, SE	Mary Free Bed Hospital & Rehabilitation Center	J. L. Doyle, M.D.
NEW JERSEY		
Atlantic City (08401) 4100 Atlantic Avenue	Children's Seashore House	Henry S. Cecil, M.D.
Longport (08403) 24th and Atlantic Avenue	Betty Bacharach Home for Afflicted Children	John M. Namee, M.D.
NEW YORK		
Bayside (11360) 20-01 126th Street	St. Mary's Hospital for Children	Charles Weyhnuller. M.D.
New York City (10003) 321 East 15th Street	New York Infirmary	Leoni N. Claman, M.D.
Valhalla (10595)	Blythedale Children's Hospital	Armond V. Mascia, M.D.

AREA SERVED		BED CAPACITY		AGE		LENGTH OF STAY		
Local	Out of State	Total	Asthma	Min.	Max.	Min.	Avg.	Max.
Yes	Yes	66	as needed		24	3 mos.	6 mos.	2 yrs.
Yes	Yes	62	10		15		85 days	
Yes	Yes	300	12	5	15	6 mos.	12 mos.	2 yrs.
Yes	Yes	86	14–19		16	2 wks.	3–4 mos.	18–24 mos.
Yes	Yes	104	as needed		18			
Yes	Yes	76	30	2	12	6 mos.	1 yr.	2 yrs.
Yes	Yes	78	as needed		10		1 yr.	2 yrs.
Yes		34	6		16	2 wks.		
Yes		100	6	2	16	6 mos.	1 yr.	2 yrs.

Institutes for the Rehabilitation of Chronic Asthma (continued)

ADDRESS	NAME OF INSTITUTE	MEDICAL DIRECTOR
OHIO		
Cincinnati (45219) 119 Wellington Place	Convalescent Hospital for Children	Joseph E. Ghory, M.D.
Cleveland (44104)	Health Hill Hospital for Children	William I. Staples, M.D.
OKLAHOMA		
Oklahoma City P.O. Box 888	Children's Convalescent Hospital	Harris Riley, M.D.
PENNSYLVANIA		
Philadelphia (19131) Conshocken Road	Children's Heart Hospital	Herbert Mansmann, M.D.
VERMONT		
Pittsford (05763)	Caverly Child Health Center	Emmett L. Fagan, M.D.
CANADA		
British Columbia	Queen Alexandra Solarium for Crippled Children	David M. Boyd, M.D.
Ontario 350 Rumsey Road (17)	Ontario Crippled Children's Center	Harold Williams, M.D.

AREA SERVED		BED CAPACITY		AGE		LENGTH OF STAY		
Local	Out of State	Total	Asthma	Min.	Max.	Min.	Avg.	Max.
Yes	Yes	100	25		18	2 wks.	3 mos.	2 yrs.
Yes	Yes	54	as needed		16		75 days	
Yes	Yes	72	as needed		20			
Yes	Yes	65	as needed		18		4 mos.	
Yes	Yes	36	as needed	2	14		18 mos.	
Yes	Prov.	68	3–12		15	6 wks.	6 mos.	2 yrs.
Yes	Prov.	105	10–15		18	3 mos.	4 mos.	5 mos.

9 Summary of the Main Allergic Disorders of Babies and Children

This summary is provided for sophisticated parents who themselves have had allergies and have become justifiably alarmed by the onset of an allergy in their child, as well as for the new parents who know nothing about allergy and find it difficult to judge how serious their child's allergy is. For both kinds of parents, a summary of the main allergic disorders, together with their treatment, gives quick, reassuring, and authoritative information.

Disease	Cause	Symptoms	Duration	Treatment
Allergy in general	Abnormal sensitivity to a food, a pollen, a dust, a mold, or a drug	Red, itchy eyes; clogged swollen, watery nose; sneezing; coughing; hives; rashes; eczema; frequent colds; hay fever; asthma; vague nervous symptoms	Until cause of sensitivity is removed	Antihistamines for nose and eye allergies; adrenalin and aminophylline for asthma attacks; desensitization for long-range treatment in inhalant allergies; steroids for refractory allergies and in life-endangering situations

Disease	Cause	Symptoms	Duration	Treatment
Asthma (immunological)	A food, an inhalant allergen, or an infection	Acute attacks of wheezing and coughing; difficult breathing	From a few minutes to a few days	Adrenalin injection for acute attacks; desensitization for long-range treatment, if cause is an inhalant; removal of the suspected allergens when possible
Colic in a bottlefed atopic baby	Allergy to milk	Onset of colic immediately after taking bottle, together with gas and irregular bowel movements	Lasts as long as baby is on milk	Milk-free diet
Bronchitis	Infection; inhalant allergens such as house dust, pollen, or foods; polluted city air; tobacco smoke	Dry nonproductive cough, with slight generalized wheezing in chest	Depends on diagnosis	Antibiotics for infection, removal of irritant or allergen; mucus-softening agents; moisture in bedroom
Conjunctivitis	Allergy to pollen or molds; air pollution; infection	Red, itchy, and tearing eyes	Depends on cause	Eye drops; antihistamine by mouth for itch; desensitization for long-range treatment of allergy

Disease	Cause	Symptoms	Duration	Treatment
Croup	Postnasal drip, which irritates the vocal cords by dripping on them	Appears in children under 5 years of age; sudden onset without fever; barking cough; difficult breathing as child goes to bed	Lasts ½ to 3 hours	Cold steam in room from vaporizer; call doctor immediately, as this condition may require hospitalization
Diaper rash	Sensitivity to soap, detergents, or rubber pants; irritation from urine and stool	Onset in early months and mostly during hot weather; appears as red pimples over itchy skin; diapers have odor of ammonia	Depends on type of treatment	Use mild soap; eliminate bleaches, detergents, and rubber pants; boil diapers or use disposable ones; expose area to air as much as possible
Eczema	Food or inhalant allergy; irritating material coming in contact with the skin	Rash and red patches on folds of arms, knees, and on cheeks starting in early months of life	Clears naturally in third or fourth year of life or may remain for many years later	Remove allergenic foods or contactants; use special soap and lotion to soothe the inflamed skin
Hay fever	Allergy to a pollen or to molds	Disease recurs strictly on a seasonal basis, as stuffed-up, itchy, and running nose with red, watery, itchy eyes	Depends on treatment	Antihistamines for symptomatic relief; desensitization for a more permanent and prolonged relief, and also to avoid complications

Disease	Cause	Symptoms	Duration	Treatment
Hives	Allergy to foods, drugs, bacteria; emotional upheaval; exposure to heat, cold, or physical pressure	Itchy wheals on different parts of the skin	Wheals last a few hours to a few days	Remove cause; treat emotional stress; soothing baths and lotions for symptomatic relief
Food intolerance	Indigestion, contaminated food, allergy to a food	Vomiting, constipation, diarrhea, colic, gas, canker sores in mouth, skin rashes	Depends on cause	Elimination of implicated food
Insect and bee stings	Allergy to venom of the bee or insect	Appear from ½ minute to a few hours after the sting as a local swelling with itching or anaphylactic shock	Depends on intensity of allergy and place of bite or sting	Adrenalin injections for shock, antihistamines for itching, long-range treatment with desensitization, prevention with ingestion of vitamin B₁ during summer
Poison ivy	Allergy to the oil coating of the plant	Appears a few hours after contact with the plant as an itchy rash, followed later by watery blisters	Depends upon the intensity of the allergy, the age of the child, and the frequency of the exposure to the plant	Symptomatic, depending on the stage in which the disease is first seen; extreme cases may require corticosteroids

10 Prescribing for the Atopic Child

Medicine is not only a science; it is also an art. It does not consist of compounding pills and plasters; it deals with the very processes of life, which must be understood before they may be guided.   Paracelsus

THE PSYCHOSOMATIC APPROACH

Psychological factors seem to influence the drug and desensitization response of children who suffer from atopic eczema, asthma, migraine headaches, and chronic hives. Even though emotional pathology does not initiate any of these illnesses, it can influence both their course and the outcome of their treatment. The effect of a drug would then differ according to the mood and circumstances of the atopic child who is using it.

Kinds of Reactions to a Drug

Drugs prescribed to atopic children usually work in a predictable fashion. Sometimes they do not do so because the child reacts to them in his own way. A reaction is an unanticipated response to a drug. A definition of a few common reactions to drugs gives a clear picture of their nature.

1. Toxicity. This is a drug reaction caused by an overdosage. It is predictable, constant, and avoidable. An example is a coma after taking too many sleeping pills.

2. Intolerance. This is caused by an increase in the expected response to a drug. An example is extreme lowering of the temperature of a baby after a usual dose of aspirin.

3. Side effect. This is an undesirable, yet unavoidable side action of a drug. An example is sleepiness while using antihistamines.

4. Secondary effect. This is a by-product of a primary action of a drug. An example is a fungus infection after a prolonged use of antibiotics.

5. Allergy. This is synonymous with hypersensitivity. It is an immunological reaction to a drug. An example is hives after using penicillin.

ALLERGY TO DRUGS PRESCRIBED IN PEDIATRIC PRACTICE

Drug allergy is less severe in children than in adults. Drugs sensitize when first used, and open the door later on to dangerous allergic reactions. Any drug can cause allergy, but some drugs cause it more frequently and more dangerously than others. Because there is no sure way to test for drug sensitivity, we have to keep an exact record of all the known drug allergies of a child so that he can avoid them in the future. This is especially important in case of allergy to penicillin or to aspirin.

Clinically, a drug allergy may be suspected if it meets these criteria: (1) the reaction does not resemble the usual action of the drug; (2) an incubation period exists during which the drug is well-tolerated; (3) a minute amount of the drug can precipitate the whole symptom complex of the allergic picture.

The diagnosis of a drug allergy must be clinical, because skin testing for drugs has little value (except for patch tests in contact dermatitis), and a provocative challenge by another dose of the drug is too dangerous to perform.

The symptoms of allergy to drugs are fever, serum sickness, anaphylaxis, blood diseases (hemolytic anemia, purpura, and so forth), and skin eruptions such as hives, erythema, photosensitization, and jaundice.

To prevent these allergic reactions, the parents must familiarize themselves thoroughly with one or two drugs of each class used in the treatment of their child and ignore the vast number of other drugs about which they are less knowledgeable. In general, they are better off using old and familiar drugs, where unexpected allergy is not likely to happen. Also, they should not push their doctor to try a new drug they have heard about until the benefits, the side effects, and the allergic reactions to the drug become so well known and established as to warrant the risk in trying it. Furthermore, they should guard against using a drug longer than necessary, and adapt the dosage of the medicine to the needs of their own particular child, because undertreatment or overtreatment may result if the age of the child, his particular sensitivities, and his peculiar constitution are not taken into consideration. In general, the most parents can offer their child is some symptomatic relief. However, symptom suppression must not delay appropriate attention to underlying causes. In allergy, skin testing and specific desensitization still remain a cardinal point in the treatment of an allergic child.

DRUGS FREQUENTLY PRESCRIBED FOR THE ALLERGIC CHILD

The Importance of Water

Water forms 60 percent of our weight, transports our foods and waste, helps to regulate our temperature, and softens our mucus to facilitate its expulsion. There are many ways to supply the lungs with water. One is to eat foods that contain water. Another is to drink Coke, milk, soups, and so forth. A third way is with steam inhalation with a cold-air or hot-air vaporizer. A fourth way is to add a potent automatically regulated vaporizer to the central heating system of the house.

Cough Syrups

Coughing is the child's response to an irritation anywhere in the respiratory tract, and it may have any one of a number of causes. Its most frequent cause is a viral infection or the common cold. This kind of cough usually responds to home remedies, such as hot drinks, aspirin, and steam inhalation. However, if the cough becomes worse and lasts more than two or three days, the child should have some sort of medication, such as an antibiotic plus a standard cough syrup to which antihistamines have been added. We have to make sure, however, that the cough syrup does not contain any codeine which suppresses the cough. The antihistamine is added to the cough syrup on the assumption that it will relieve the bronchial spasm as well as the swelling of the respiratory mucosa. Also, antihistamines in general have a calming effect on the nervous system, and therefore allay the anxiety that goes along with the cough.

If a cough has become chronic, we must look either for smoke and air pollution—which may have caused a sinusitis, chronic bronchitis, or emphysema—or for an allergy. Besides eliminating or treating the causes, we prescribe, in all cases, drops of potassium iodide to soften the mucus and facilitate expectoration. There are many ways to prescribe this useful medication, one of which is to start with one drop in a teaspoonful of milk four times daily, to be increased by one drop each day. Example:

> One drop four times daily first day
> Two drops four times daily second day
> Three drops four times daily third day . . .
> Seven drops four times daily seventh day

until ten drops four times daily is reached, then diminished to one drop per day. Example:

Nine drops four times daily eleventh day
Eight drops four times daily twelfth day
Seven drops four times daily thirteenth day . . .
One drop four times daily twentieth day.

This process of increasing and diminishing drops should be continued for a period of three months. The drops of potassium iodide may cause a brassy and burning feeling in the mouth and throat, soreness of the gums, increased salivation, skin rashes, and occasionally goiter. All these side effects disappear within a few days after stopping medication, except for goiter, which may last up to two months.

Antihistamines

This is a group of drugs that has acquired a definite place in the treatment of allergic disorders. Even though antihistamines do not cure allergies, they give symptomatic relief to many of their manifestations. They are best used in seasonal and perennial allergic rhinitis, vasomotor rhinitis, allergic conjunctivitis due to inhalant allergens and foods, and in uncomplicated allergic skin manifestations of urticaria and angioedema.

Antihistamines should not be given to newborns or premature infants, to nursing mothers, or to people suffering from lower respiratory infections, glaucoma, stenotic peptic ulcers, bladder neck obstruction, and duodenal obstruction.

When given in large quantities, antihistamines cause hallucinations, convulsions, diminished alertness, excitation, possible malformations in the fetuses of pregnant women, and even death.

The side effects of antihistamines are sedation, sleepiness, dryness of the mouth, thickening of the bronchial secretions, dizziness, epigastric distress, and disturbed coordination. Because of these side effects, anyone using antihistamines should not engage in mechanical operations requiring alertness.

The following is a list of antihistamines in common usage: Benadryl, Clistin, Co-Pyronil, Dimetane, Disomer, Forhistal, Phenergan, Polarmine, Pyribenzamine, Teldrin, and Histadyl. Some antihistamines come mixed with decongestants: Actifed, Demazin, Dimetapp, Ornade, and Triaminic.

Hormones

Because we live in an era in which computers have been made to replace doctors' brains, research is being geared to manufacture drugs that cure symptoms, not illnesses. The old precept that a doctor has to find the cause of an illness in order to cure it is slowly being replaced by a facile dependence on symptomatic relief brought about by the use of potent drugs. In allergy, this is being achieved with hormones derived from the suprarenal and pituitary glands. These are "miracle" or lifesaving drugs when used properly, and very dangerous if used indiscriminately. Twenty years of experience in the use of these drugs has shown that they do not cure allergy, but only mask its symptoms. Furthermore, their side effects are often so serious that the trouble they create becomes more important than the disease they are supposed to cure. This happens because hormones act not only on their target cells, but on a wide variety of body organs as well. Some of these side effects are disturbances in the sodium and potassium balance of the blood; the breakdown of tissue proteins; the mobilization of fats, sugars, and carbohydrates. That is why any child who must use corticosteroids or ACTH should be checked for low blood pressure, weight increase, depression, abnormal growth, sugar in the urine, and hairiness. In all cases, hormones are to be used as sparingly as possible because their use brings about an addiction to them caused by a shrinking in the size of the suprarenal gland. Furthermore, they should not be prescribed to children who have an antibiotic-resistant inflammation; however, their dosage should be increased in a child who is due for surgery.

The main commercial adrenal corticosteroids are the following: Meticorten, Aristocort, Medrol, Decadron, Celestone, Hydrocortisone, Meticortelone, Cortef, Kenalog. Some of these preparations are incorporated in pastes to apply on skin afflicted with eczema or contact dermatitis.

The dramatic relief of symptoms brought about by the use of these drugs has led to inordinate publicity on their use. However, experience and time have challenged their indiscriminate usage, but have assigned to them a place of great importance in the lifesaving emergency treatment of intractable asthma. As such, they cannot be replaced, but under no circumstances should they be used to substitute for a proper diagnosis of an allergic disorder, or for its treatment with desensitization.

Tranquilizers

In childhood, only the "minor tranquilizers" or the antianxiety drugs should be prescribed. These are Meprobamate, Atarax, Vistaril, Librium, and Valium. Two allergic conditions may require their use: extreme anxiety in asthma cases, and constant itching in cases of eczema. For the latter, Atarax or Vistaril is the drug of choice.

Antibiotics

These drugs control infections, but some calamities from their misuse may occur. Many antibiotics are incorporated in over-the-counter sprays, lozenges, and troches for use with sore throats. An atopic child should never use such preparations because he may become sensitive to them and have allergic reactions when he really needs them. If a child has an infection that warrants antibiotics, then they should be given to him in adequate dosage and for an appropriate period of time. No haphazard, halfhearted, over-the-counter prescription will do. Furthermore, many infections are due to viruses, and these do not respond to antibiotics. Viruses, however, lower the resistance of the mucosa, and allow the regular bacteria that lie on its surface to seep underneath, where they multiply and cause a secondary bacterial infection. By prescribing an antibiotic for a viral infection, we eliminate a good tool to fight off a subsequent bacterial infection.

Allergic reactions to antibiotics occur more frequently in atopic children than in others, and more readily if the drug has been given by injection and not by mouth. This is especially true in the use of penicillin, which must not be prescribed for an atopic child except when absolutely needed.

Other reactions to antibiotics include a sore mouth, cramps in the stomach, vomiting, diarrhea, and a generalized rash with a rectal itch. Such reactions frequently occur after the use of tetracyclines and may result in the suppression of bacteria normally found in the gastrointestinal tract. The normal intestine contains various bacteria, each of which inhibits the overabundant growth of the others. When this balance is upset by an antibiotic therapy meant to destroy one kind of germ, an overgrowth of the other types of germs takes place, manifesting itself by the symptoms mentioned above. To counterbalance them the parent should feed the child yogurt, which is nothing but a culture of bacteria in milk. It replaces those bacteria which have been destroyed, and restores a normal balance among the various types of bacteria that dwell in the intestines. It is a healthy food for the child, because it resembles cow's milk in its content of protein, fat, carbohydrates, vitamins, minerals, and calories. Some of its brands contain no fat, and these are useful in the treatment of diarrhea. Yogurt feeding is currently being used in the treatment of various intestinal disturbances in Bulgaria, Turkey, and the Middle East, and deserves a try in the gastrointestinal disturbances caused by antibiotics.

A few antibiotics are very toxic, and their use must be limited. Examples are streptomycin, which may cause deafness, and chloromycetin, which may injure the bone marrow irreversibly.

These are the antibiotics in common use:

1. Penicillin, which should not be used for an atopic child; if absolutely necessary, use it by mouth and not by injection. Never use an ointment that contains it.

2. Tetracycline, Panalba, Signemycin—all broad spectrum anti-

biotics. Guard against monilial superinfection while using them.

3. Streptomycin and Chloromycetin—not to be used, except under strict medical prescription and supervision.

Penicillin

This is one of the least toxic drugs from the point of view of its dosage, yet allergy to it is a very serious illness. Allergy to penicillin depends on the amount given, the route of its administration, the prior exposure of the child to it, its location, and whether infections and other diseases are present during its usage. The incidence of penicillin allergy among the child population of this country may be judged only approximately, as only its spectacular reactions are noticed, while minor symptoms may be overlooked and confused with the disease being treated.

One type of penicillin allergy is the immediate one. This occurs a few minutes after its injection or ingestion, and ranges from a mild fever to itching, rashes, hives, serum sickness, asthma, hemorrhage, contact dermatitis, or even anaphylactic shock—although this last is rare in children. Penicillin sensitizes only at an early age, but it does open the door for major allergies later.

Another type of reaction is the accelerated one. This occurs two to three days after contact and manifests itself as hives, laryngeal edema, or a choking sensation. A third type of reaction is the delayed one, manifesting itself as a serum sickness type of allergy three or four days after its use. Lastly, there sometimes is a very delayed reaction, which occurs one week after contact, and manifests itself as a rash, hemolytic anemia, or pains in the joints.

Children who have had no previous contact with penicillin may show sensitivity reactions if they drink milk from cows treated with penicillin, or eat moldy food, or are given their immunizations with syringes previously used to inject penicillin. Boiling and sterilization do not destroy penicillin or prevent allergy to it.

The present allergy tests for penicillin sensitivity are useful, but have limited value. If negative they cannot be taken to exclude sensitivity to penicillin, while if positive they do not mean that the child will always react adversely to it.

Aspirin

Acetyl salicylic acid, better known as aspirin, may cause all or one of the following allergic symptoms: hives, perennial rhinitis, polyposis, bronchial asthma. The other salicylates, even though very similar in structure to aspirin, do not cause allergic symptoms.

We do not know how aspirin causes allergic symptoms. It is probable that the small molecule of aspirin unites with a bigger molecule found in the body of the child to form a large molecule called a *hapten*. It is this large molecule that is capable of causing allergies, and knowledge of its composition would have to precede any immunological test done to detect sensitivity to aspirin. So far, we do not know enough about the composition of the hapten to enable us to make a test to detect it.

Drugs Used in Dentistry

Dentists, as well as parents of atopic children, usually show undue concern before a dental work-up about possible sensitivities to local anesthetics or tooth-filling material. Although allergy to all of these drugs is theoretically possible, it is most unusual. Reactions to local anesthetics are very frequently psychogenic, or result from an accidental injection of the material directly into the blood. To diagnose an allergy to these drugs we have to inject them subcutaneously in very small amounts to observe the reaction they may provoke. A skin testing for these drugs is of no value. Even though there is no 100 percent allergy-proof drug to use in dentistry, allergy to a regional anesthetic is very rare. These drugs are to be assumed safe drugs, unless known to be otherwise because of a previous reaction.

Drugs Used in Anesthesia for an Asthmatic Child

Before being given any kind of anesthesia for an operation, an asthmatic child must check into the hospital two to three days before that operation so he can spend these days in an allergy-free bedroom (St. Vincent's Hospital of the City of New York has a very elaborate one). Furthermore, if the child needs antibiotics or corticosteroids to prepare him for the operation, these have to be given two days in advance to give them a chance to work.

A good rule is to start the anesthesia with diazepam or pentothal and follow this by halothane, because this drug has a bronchodilator action. The anesthetist must give the gas to the child, using a mask rather than intubation, and the gas given must be humidified and heated to 37° C., and kept at that level all during the administration of the anesthesia to prevent bronchospasm. The child's hospital room must also be properly heated and humidified.

11 Preparing Special Diets and Cooking for the Allergic Child

GENERAL NOTES ON FOOD FOR ALLERGY-FREE DIETS

Allergic children, like all children, like colorful foods, foods free of tough fibers, seeds, or stones, and finger foods that are in strips and can be easily picked up and eaten. But their food must not only be adequate from the caloric point of view, but acceptable to them socially; that is, it must not embarrass them when they eat it in company or in school.

The foods suggested in this chapter—which do not have to be prepared fresh each time, but can be frozen and stored—are suitable for any age group, and the information given will provide a basis for modifying some of your own favorite recipes. (In addition, we have included at the end of the chapter a list of publications containing allergy-free recipes.) All the ingredients given are hypoallergenic, and should not cause problems. However, should any recipe contain a food known to cause an allergy for the intended user, this food should be replaced by another one. For instance, if the troublemaker is chocolate, try butterscotch or vanilla. The nuts called for in these recipes are not essential, and can be replaced by raisins or dried fruits.

In shopping for prepared foods, from baby foods through crackers, cookies, and other commercially baked products, read the labels carefully. You will discover that many products are made, for example, without wheat, eggs, or milk—sometimes without all three. Careful label reading will also enable you to avoid the other, more uncommon foods to which your child may be allergic. The parents must keep the list below and mark on it the foods to which their child is allergic, adding any other such foods that are not already included.

Dairy Products	Fruits	Cereals
( ) Milk	( ) Oranges	( ) Buckwheat
( ) Cream	( ) Bananas	( ) Wheat
( ) Margarine	( ) Strawberries	( ) Corn
( ) Ice Cream	( ) Lemons	( ) Barley
( ) Cheese	( ) Grapefruit	( ) Rye
( ) Butter	( ) Peaches	( ) Rice
	( ) Apples	

Vegetables	Poultry, Fish, Eggs, Meat	Miscellaneous
( ) Onions	( ) Beef	( ) Coffee
( ) Celery	( ) Chicken	( ) Tea
( ) Potatoes	( ) Pork	( ) Colas
( ) Peas	( ) Fish	( ) Chocolate
( ) Beans	( ) Shellfish	( ) Vanilla
( ) Tomatoes	( ) Veal	( ) Nuts
( ) Corn	( ) Lamb	( ) Spices
( ) Cabbage	( ) Eggs	( ) Garlic
( ) Lettuce		

Food Additives as a Cause of Child Allergy

The use of artificially preserved foods in the diets of allergic children entails some hazards because of additives. Additives are (1) dyes derived from coal tar, plants, or animals; (2) preservatives derived from chemicals, such as sodium benzoate, lactic acid, and citric acid; (3) emulsifiers and thickeners, such as karaya gum,

gum arabic, or tragacanth, (4) spices and condiments, such as mustard, pepper, ginger, cinnamon, cloves, nutmeg, vanilla or almonds; (5) linseed and peanuts, which may be inadvertently present in the milk of cows that have been fed these foods; (6) antibotics such as penicillin, and hormones such as estrogens, which may also be present in the milk of cows that needed to be treated with these drugs.

Additives are incorporated into foods during their production, storage, and processing. Their importance in causing allergic symptoms is extremely great because more than half of the food a child eats is ready to cook and may have additives. The other half only is fresh and ready to eat.

Some patterns of allergic and neurological behaviors are now frequently being encountered in children, and they are thought of as being caused by additives.

Respiratory. Allergic rhinitis, nasal polyps, cough, edema of the vocal cords, asthma.

Skin. Itching, dermographism, urticaria, angioedema.

Gastrointestinal. Flatulence and gas, constipation, chancres in the mouth.

Neurologic. Headaches, behavioral disturbances. Behavioral disturbances are perhaps the most important and the most dramatic of all the adverse reactions caused by additives. These manifest themselves as restlessness, hyperactivity, decreased attention span, and a complete disruption of the normal life at home and in school. At home the children are stubborn, hostile, and rebellious. At school they are disruptive, in conflict with their schoolmates, and show learning difficulties in spite of high IQs.

Food planning for a growing population of children that is first bottlefed, and then given already prepared foods, has become more and more dependent upon synthetic food products, most of which are flavored and colored with artificial additives. This creates for the growing child population of the world an unprecedented problem, one that needs curbing through legislation.

ALLERGY-FREE DIETS

The Milk-Free Diet

Milk sensitivity varies in intensity. Some children cannot tolerate milk in any form; others can tolerate it dried or evaporated; still others can tolerate goat's milk only and not cow's milk. Milk-sensitive children must avoid milk and all its derivatives.

Milk is consumed as cow's milk—fresh, dry, evaporated, or condensed—or is incorporated in:

1. Beverages, such as chocolate milk, hot cocoa, or any beverage made with milk.
2. Breads, those commercial breads or rolls that have milk added to the ingredients, and zwieback.
3. Butter.
4. Cheese.
5. Cookies and cakes.
6. Cream, including whipped cream and sour cream, cream sauces, creamed soups, creamed vegetables, milk gravy, milk chowder.
7. Desserts, such as cream pies, custards, ice cream, sherbet; and candy, such as chocolate or caramel.
8. Mashed potatoes.
9. Meats, such as meat loaf, cold cuts, frankfurters, and so forth.

In preparing milk-free meals, besides the specifically milk-free recipes that are given here, on pages 188–222, any standard recipe that does not include milk can be used safely. And milk-free margarine (like Mazola) or vegetable shortenings in liquid or solid form (such as Crisco, Spry, or Snowdrift) can be used in place of butter in most recipes—and of course the milk-free margarine can be used in place of butter as a spread. Also, many commercial breads and crackers are milk free, as are most of the gelatin and fruit desserts. Variety can be added to the milk-free diet by the use of nondairy whipped toppings (such as Rich's) and creamers, but their labels should be checked carefully because a number of products contain sodium caseinate, which is a milk derivative. Below is a listing of Nabisco products that do not contain milk or milk products. For milk-free baby foods by Beech-Nut and Heinz, see pages 227–245.

Brazil nut cookies
Brownie thin wafers

Chipsters potato snacks
chocolate chip snaps
chocolate covered grahams
chocolate Pinwheels cakes
chocolate snaps
cinnamon graham treats
Comet cones
Comet cups
Comet pilot cones
Cookie Break vanilla
   flavored creme sandwich
Cookie Break vanilla wafers
Cream of Wheat cereal—
   instant mix 'n eat, quick,
   regular
Crown pilot crackers

Dairy wafers round
Dandy soup and oyster
   crackers
Dromedary corn bread mix
Dromedary corn muffin
Dromedary dates
Dromedary gingerbread mix

family favorites pecan drop
   cookies
French onion crackers

Nabisco graham cracker
   crumbs
Nabisco graham crackers
Gem soup and chili crackers

Nabisco iced fruit cookies
Nabisco iced oatmeal raisin
   cookies

lemon jumble rings
lemon snaps

Meal Mates sesame bread
   wafers
Mister Salty pretzel rings
Mister Salty 3-ring pretzels
Mister Salty veri-thin
   pretzels
Mister Salty veri-thin
   pretzel sticks

Nabisco 100% bran
Nabisco rice honeys
Nabisco salted peanuts
Nabisco shredded wheat
Wheat Honeys cereals

old fashion ginger snaps
Oysterettes soup and oyster
   crackers

Nabisco pecan shortbread
   cookies

Premium crackers unsalted
tops
Premium saltine crackers
Pretzelettes

Ritz crackers

Sociables crackers
Soup Mates tiny soup
crackers
Nabisco spiced wafers
Spoon Size shredded wheat
sugar Honey Maid graham
crackers

Team flakes
Triangle Thins crackers
Triscuit wafers

Uneeda biscuit unsalted
tops

vanilla crumbs
Veri-Thin pretzel sticks

Waverly wafers
wheat thins crackers

Zu-Zu ginger snaps

The Cereal-Free Diet

The members of the cereal family are wheat, rice, rye, oats, barley, malt, and corn. A child who is sensitive to two types of cereal grains must avoid the whole family. These foods contain cereals:

1. Beverages, such as flavored milk drinks (malted, chocolate, etc.), instant coffee unless 100% coffee, coffee substitutes, beer, gin, whiskey.
2. Bread, such as commercial breads including rye, soy, cracked wheat, graham, whole wheat, corn bread which usually contains wheat flour, Matzoh, pretzels, melba toast, zwieback.
3. Cereals, either dry or cooked.
4. Crackers and cookies. All commercial cookies, even arrowroot, contain some wheat.
5. Desserts, such as cakes, doughnuts, pastries, ice cream cones, commercial ice cream, prepared mixes for cakes and cookies, commercial pie fillings (which are generally thickened with wheat flour).
6. Gravies, sauces, or cream soups. Commercially canned soups are usually prepared with wheat flour.

7. Macaroni, noodles, spaghetti, and other pasta products.

8. Meats, including those breaded or prepared with wheat flour; cold cuts such as bologna, wieners, and some sausages; canned meat dishes with sauces such as chili.

9. Pancakes and waffles, unless made from special recipes. Commercial mixes, including buckwheat, may contain some wheat.

10. Miscellaneous foods include cream cheese dips, seasoned potato chips, soy sauce, salad dressings, commercial baked beans.

Try to select recipes for cereal-free breads, cakes, biscuits, and so forth, that are adaptable to your needs and can be modified when necessary.

If you wish to substitute flours while baking or making gravies, the following is a list of equivalents. Keep in mind that rice flour is to be given preference over all others, since it is hypoallergenic. One cup of wheat flour is equivalent to:

1 cup barley flour
⅞ cup rice flour
1¼ cups rye flour
1⅓ cups oat flour
⅝ cup potato starch flour

For thickening gravies, sauces, and puddings, 1 tablespoon of wheat flour is equivalent to:

½ tablespoon potato starch
½ tablespoon arrowroot starch
1 tablespoon rice flour
2 teaspoons quick-cooking tapioca

On a wheat-free diet, some products are easier to get commercially. These include rice cereal (Rice Chex, Rice Krispies), rye wafers (Ry Krisp), and corn meal (Corn Chex, Corn Flakes).

For a listing of wheat-free baby foods by Beech-Nut and Heinz, see pages 227–245.

Following is a listing of some of the Nabisco products that do not contain wheat:

cheese flavored Flings curls	Nabisco rice honeys
Chipsters potato snacks	Nabisco salted peanuts
Corn Diggers snacks	Shapies cheese flavored dip
Dromedary dates	delights
Dromedary fudge and frost-	Shapies cheese flavored
ing mix	shells
Dromedary pimientos	Snack Mate pasteurized
Korkers corn chips	process cheese spreads

The Chicago Dietetic Supply, Inc., markets a grainless mix, Cellu Grainless Mix, well suited to substitute for cereals in baking breads and biscuits. This mix is especially prepared for use in diets that forbid cereal grains of any origin. The ingredients of Cellu Grainless Mix are potato starch, soybean flour, soybean shortening, cane sugar, phosphate of calcium, sodium bicarbonate, and salt.

Wheat-free recipes other than the ones included in this chapter (pages 188–222) may be obtained from the sources listed on pages 225–226.

The Egg-Free Diet

Egg should be carefully avoided by the allergic child. These foods contain egg:

1. Beverages, such as eggnog, root beer, malted drinks, and any prepared drinks made with eggs or egg powder.
2. Breads and rolls, including those with glazed crusts, sweet rolls, pancakes, waffles, doughnuts, pretzels, French toast.
3. Broth.
4. Cookies and cakes.
5. Desserts, such as cream pies, meringues, custards, ice cream, sherbet, some candy.
6. Noodles.

7. Meats, such as meat loaf, meat balls, croquettes, breaded meats.
8. Salad dressings and mayonnaise, egg sauces such as hollandaise.

Egg-free recipes other than the ones included in this chapter (pages 188–222) may be obtained from the sources listed on page 226. For a listing of egg-free baby foods by Beech-Nut and Heinz, see pages 227–245.

Some Nabisco foods that do not contain egg or egg products are listed below:

Appeteasers tiny crackers, crescent-roll-shaped
Appeteasers tiny crackers ham tasting/shaped
Appeteasers tiny onion shaped/flavored

bacon flavored thin crackers
Bali Hai Hawaiian flavor creme sandwich
Barnum's Animal crackers
Biscos sugar wafers
Biscos waffles
Brazil nut cookies
brown edge wafers
Brownie thin wafers
Brownie thin wafers vanilla flavored
butter flavored thins crackers
butter flavored sesame snack crackers

Cameo creme sandwich
cheese cracker small

cheese cracker square
cheese flavored Flings curls
cheese 'n bacon flavored sandwich
cheese Nips crackers
cheese-on-rye sandwich
cheese peanut butter sandwich variety pack
cheese sandwich
cheese Tid-Bits crackers
Chicken in a Biskit crackers
Chippers potato crackers
Chips Ahoy! chocolate chip cookies
Chipsters potato snacks
chocolate chip cookies
chocolate chip snacks
chocolate covered grahams
chocolate crumbs
chocolate Pinwheels cakes
chocolate snaps
cinnamon graham treats
cocoanut bars cookies
Comet pilot cones

Cookie Break assorted
fudge creme sandwich
Cookie Break chocolate
fudge creme sandwich
Cookie Break sugar wafers
Corn Diggers snack
Cowboys and Indians
cookies
Cream of Wheat cereals,
instant mix 'n eat, quick,
regular
creme wafer sticks
Crown peanut bars
Crown pilot crackers

dairy wafers round
Dandy soup and oyster
crackers
Doo Dads snacks
Dromedary banana nut roll
Dromedary chocolate nut
roll
Dromedary cornbread mix
Dromedary corn muffin mix
Dromedary date nut roll
Dromedary fudge and frost-
ing mix
Dromedary orange nut roll
Dromedary pimientos
Dromedary pound cake

Escort crackers

Family Favorites chocolate
chip cookies
Family Favorites chocolate
nut cookies

Family Favorites raisin buns
cookies
French onion cracker
fudge creme sandwich
cookies
Gem soup and chili crackers
graham cracker crumbs
graham crackers
ice fruit cookies
Ideal chocolate peanut logs

Hey Days caramel peanut
logs

lemon snaps

Mallowmars chocolate
cakes
malted milk peanut butter
sandwich
marshmallow puffs
marshmallow Twirls
Meal Mates sesame bread
wafers
Melody chocolate cookies
Minarets cakes
mint sandwich cookies
Mister Salty pretzel rings
Mister Salty 3 ring pretzels
Mister Salty Veri-Thin
pretzels
Mister Salty Veri-Thin
pretzel sticks

Nabisco devil's food cakes
Nabisco fancy crest cakes
Nabisco iced fruit cookies

Nabisco iced oatmeal raisin cookies
Nabisco macaroon sandwich
Nabisco oatmeal cookies
Nabisco raisin fruit biscuit
Nabisco salted peanuts
Nabisco shredded wheat
Nabisco spiced wafers
Nabisco rice honeys

Oreo creme sandwich
O-So-Gud cheese peanut butter sandwich
Oysterettes soup and oyster crackers

Pantry grahams
peanut butter & jelly tasting patties
peanut creme patties
peanut creme sticks
Premium crackers unsalted tops
Premium saltine crackers
pretzelettes

Ritz cheese crackers
Ritz crackers

Shapies cheese flavored dip delights

Shapies cheese flavored shells
Sip'n Chips cheese flavored snacks
Snack Mates pasteurized process cheese spreads
Sociables crackers
Soup Mates tiny soup crackers
Spoon-Size shredded wheat
striped shortbread
sugar Honey Maid graham crackers
Swiss 'n ham flavored Flings curls

Team flakes
Toastettes toaster pastries
Triangle Thins crackers
Triscuit wafers
Twigs sesame/cheese flavored snack sticks

Uneeda biscuit unsalted tops

vanilla crumbs

Waverly wafers
Wheat Honey cereal
wheat thins crackers

Zu-Zu ginger snaps

SAMPLES OF ALLERGY-FREE DIET MENUS

EGG-FREE DIET MENU

Breakfast
Any kind of fruit or juice
Any kind of meat
Cereal (made without egg)
Buttered toast (made without egg)
Milk

Lunch
Vegetable soup
Cottage cheese and peaches
Jell-O
Milk

Dinner
Broiled fish
Mashed potatoes
Green beans
Salad with dressing (made without eggs)
Homemade biscuits with butter (made without eggs)
Fresh fruit
Milk

Snack
Popcorn, fruit

MILK-FREE DIET MENU

Breakfast
Orange juice
Egg
Any kind of meat
Grits

Lunch
Roast beef
Baked potato
English peas
Carrot and celery sticks
Lemonade

Dinner
Any kind of meat
Sweet potatoes with cinnamon
Spinach
Tossed salad with oil and wine vinegar
Peach tapioca
Fruit juice

CEREAL-FREE DIET MENU

Breakfast
Orange juice
Scrambled egg
Soy muffin with homemade jam
Milk

Lunch
Cold chicken
Homemade potato salad
Carrot and celery sticks
Raw apple
Milk

Dinner
Any kind of meat
Baked squash
Tossed salad with lemon juice
Peach tapioca
Apple juice

MILK-FREE, EGG-FREE DIET MENU

Breakfast
Orange juice
Toast
Jelly

Lunch
Roast beef
Baked potato
English peas
Carrot and celery sticks
Raw apple
Lemonade

Dinner
Any kind of meat
Baked squash with nutmeg
Tossed salad with oil, sugar, spice dressing
Peach tapioca
Sliced bread with jelly
Fruit juice

CEREAL-FREE, MILK-FREE DIET MENU

Breakfast
Orange juice
Soy-potato muffin with brown sugar
  or homemade jam

Lunch
Cold chicken legs
Soy-potato muffin with brown sugar
  or homemade jam
Carrot and celery sticks
Raw apple
Pineapple juice

Dinner
Any kind of meat
Baked squash with nutmeg
Tossed salad with oil, sugar, spice dressing
Peach tapioca
Soy-potato muffin with homemade jam
Apple juice

GRAIN-FREE, EGG-FREE DIET MENU

Breakfast
Orange juice
Soy-potato muffin with butter and
  brown sugar
Milk

Lunch
Yellow cheese slices
Soy-potato muffins with butter
Carrot and celery sticks
Raw apple
Milk

Dinner
Any kind of meat
Buttered baked squash with nutmeg
Tossed salad with oil, sugar, spice dressing
Peach tapioca
Soy-potato muffin with butter and homemade jam
Milk

GRAIN-FREE, MILK-FREE, EGG-FREE DIET MENU

Breakfast
Orange juice
Soy-potato muffin with brown sugar
  or homemade jam

Lunch
Cold chicken leg
Soy-potato muffin with brown sugar
  or homemade jam
Carrot and celery sticks
Raw apple
Pineapple juice

Dinner
Any kind of meat
Baked squash with nutmeg
Tossed salad with oil, sugar, spice dressing
Peach tapioca
Soy-potato muffin with cinnamon sugar
Apple juice

COOKING FOR CHILDREN WITH FOOD ALLERGIES

Cooking, especially baking, for family members allergic to wheat, eggs, or milk calls for special recipes. The recipes that follow were developed for use without some or all of these basic ingredients.

Most substitute ingredients, such as cornmeal and rolled oats, are commonly available. If others, such as rice, rye, and soybean flours, are not available at your market, they can be bought at specialty food stores.

Every recipe here has been tested for flavor, texture, and appearance of the final product. However, while the flavors of the baked products you will find here are good, the textures will not be the same as in products made with the usual ingredients. Cakes and muffins made without eggs crumble more easily than those made with eggs, and breads and cakes made with nonwheat flours will not be as light as those made with wheat flour. Also, baked products, such as muffins and biscuits, will not have that rich brown color when flours other than wheat are used. And while water may be substituted for milk in most recipes with little effect on the final product, products made without milk and eggs will require a longer baking time at a lower temperature.

Before you prepare any of these recipes, check the labels on your baking powder and shortening containers. Be sure all ingredients in these products are permitted in the diet. And note that it is better to use a hypoallergenic baking powder or a leavening agent that does not contain starch or egg white. Also, in milk-free baking, be sure you grease any pans with vegetable shortening or milk-free margarine; do not use butter. Proper storage for the foods you are preparing is important, and freezing will keep them for a very long time, provided they are wrapped properly beforehand. However, use the refrigerator for storing foods only if specified.

Finally, be sure to take note of the following table of equivalents:

60 drops	=	1 teaspoon
3 teaspoons	=	1 tablespoon
2 tablespoons	=	1 liquid ounce
4 tablespoons	=	¼ cup
16 tablespoons	=	1 cup
2 cups	=	1 pint
2 pints	=	1 quart
32 liquid ounces	=	1 quart
16 ounces	=	1 pound

Main Courses and Side Dishes

Meat Loaf I†   Serves 4 to 6

(Wheat-free, egg-free, milk-free)

  3 tablespoons instant sweet potatoes
  2 tablespoons instant chopped onion
  1 tablespoon dried parsley flakes
½ cup tomato juice (or water)
  1 pound ground beef
½ cup rice cereal crumbs or corn flake crumbs
  1 teaspoon salt
¼ teaspoon pepper

Soak the sweet potato, onion, and parsley flakes in the tomato juice for 5 minutes, then add to the meat, along with the crumbs, salt, and pepper. Mix thoroughly. Pat into a 9 x 5-inch loaf pan and bake in a preheated 350° oven for 45 minutes.

Meat Loaf II†   Serves 4 to 6

(Wheat-free, egg-free, milk-free)

½ cup prepared instant mashed potatoes, prepared with all water, no butter
  1 pound ground beef
  2 tablespoons instant chopped onion
  1 teaspoon salt
¼ teaspoon pepper

Thoroughly combine all the ingredients, then bake according to the instructions for Meat Loaf I.

The recipes in this chapter marked * have been adapted, with some revisions, from U.S. Department of Agriculture *Home and Garden Bulletin No. 147,* as has the introductory material on page 186. The recipes marked †, and those marked ‡, have been adapted, with some revisions, from material provided by The American Dietetic Association (Chicago, Illinois) and Chicago Dietetic Supply, Inc., respectively.

Oven-Fried Chicken† Serves 4 to 6

(Wheat-free, egg-free, milk-free)

2½ pounds chicken, cut into serving pieces
¼ cup salad oil
  Salt and pepper
1 cup finely crushed crisp rice or corn cereal, potato chips (4 cups before crushing), or rice flour

Rub each piece of chicken with oil, then sprinkle with salt and pepper and roll in crushed crumbs or rice flour. Arrange in a greased shallow baking dish or sheet, leaving space between the pieces. Cover tightly with foil. Bake in a preheated 400° oven for 45 minutes, or until chicken is tender. Uncover for the last 15 minutes to brown the chicken.

Barley Mushroom Casserole† Serves 8

(Wheat-free, egg-free, milk-free)

2 beef bouillon cubes
1 quart boiling water
¼ cup salad oil
2 tablespoons instant chopped onion
1 two-and-one-half-ounce can mushroom pieces
1 can pearl barley
1 teaspoon salt

Dissolve the bouillon cubes in the boiling water. Combine the oil, onions, mushrooms, and barley in an ungreased 2 quart casserole. Stir in the bouillon and salt and bake, uncovered, in a preheated 350° oven for 1 hour, stirring several times. Cover and bake 30 more minutes.

Note: This is excellent served with broiled or roasted meat.

Breads

Rye Bread† Makes 2 loaves

(Wheat-free, egg-free, milk-free)

6 cups rye flour, approximately
1 tablespoon salt
2 packages active dry yeast
½ cup instant potato flakes
2 cups hot water
½ cup molasses or granulated sugar
¼ cup salad oil

In a large bowl, thoroughly mix 2 cups of the rye flour with the salt and undissolved yeast. In a separate bowl, add the potato flakes to the hot water and whip lightly with a fork. Combine the potato-water mixture, molasses, and oil and add to the dry ingredients. Beat for 2 minutes at medium speed, scraping the bowl occasionally, then add 2 more cups flour and beat at high speed for 2 minutes, scraping the bowl occasionally. Stir in the remaining 2 cups flour, or enough to make a stiff dough.

Sprinkle a bread board with rye flour. Turn the dough out and knead until smooth and elastic (8 to 10 minutes). Place the dough in a greased bowl, cover, and let rise in a warm place until doubled in bulk (1½ to 2 hours). Punch the dough down and shape into 2 loaves. Place in 2 greased 9 x 5-inch loaf pans, cover, and let rise until doubled in bulk (30 to 45 minutes).

Bake in a preheated 350° oven for 40 minutes, or until the loaves sound hollow when tapped lightly.

BANANA RYE BREAD

Before baking this bread, the United Fruit Company, which advocates the use of it, advises reading the following questions and answers:

Q. Why is Banana Rye Bread especially suitable for persons allergic to eggs, wheat, or milk?

A. Because it is made without eggs, wheat, milk or their products.

Q. What kind of flour is used?

A. Rye flour only is used. Rye flour is marketed in four general grades—light, medium, straight, and dark. The light rye flour makes the best loaf, although the medium and straight grades can also be used. The dark rye flour is not suitable for this recipe.

Q. Where can the proper grade of rye flour be purchased?

A. From a local baker if your grocer does not carry it.

Q. Are the light, medium, and straight rye flours used in the same amounts?

A. Yes. The recipe is satisfactory for any of these three rye flours.

Q. What leavening is used?

A. Yeast (active dry or compressed).

Q. What kind of shortening is used?

A. Any kind, though butter should be avoided when there is an allergy due to milk or milk products.

Q. How ripe should the bananas be for this bread?

A. Fully ripe—yellow peel flecked with brown. Only fully ripe bananas give the bread its delicious, distinctive flavor.

Q. What is the easiest way to mash bananas?

A. Peel the bananas and slice them into a bowl. Beat with a fork, rotary egg beater, or electric mixer until liquefied and creamy. Mash the bananas just before using them.

Q. Is any special technique required in making Banana Rye Bread?

A. Yes, always grease your hands before the kneading process to facilitate manipulating the dough. Do not fail to do this, because rye flour makes a more sticky and less elastic dough than wheat flour.

Q. Does Banana Rye Bread keep well?

A. Yes. Bananas not only add flavor but help to keep the bread fresh and moist. When the bread is thoroughly cooled, store it in a clean, well-aired, covered container in a cool, dry place.

Q. How can Banana Rye Bread be used?

A. As a plain bread or for sandwiches. Makes unusually good toast.

Banana Rye Bread   Makes 2 loaves

(Wheat-free, egg-free, milk-free)

  2 packages active dry yeast
¼ cup warm (not hot) water
  1 tablespoon salt
1½ tablespoons sugar
  3 tablespoons melted vegetable shortening or vegetable oil
2¼ cups mashed ripe bananas (5 to 6 bananas)
5½ to 6 cups rye flour

Dissolve the yeast in the water and set aside. In a large bowl, mix together the salt, sugar, shortening, and bananas. Add three cups of the flour and beat until smooth, then beat in the dissolved yeast. Add 2½ cups flour gradually and mix well. Place the dough on a floured board, adding just enough additional rye flour to prevent sticking—about 6 tablespoons.

Knead lightly for about 4 minutes, then place the dough in a lightly greased bowl. Cover and let rise in a warm place until doubled in bulk (about 2 hours). Turn out again on a floured board (2 to 3 tablespoons flour) and knead lightly for about 2 minutes.

Grease the bottoms only of 2 bread pans (8 x 4 x 3 inches). Shape the dough into 2 loaves and place in the pans. Cover and let rise again in a warm place until doubled in bulk (about 1 hour). Bake in a hot oven (425°) for 5 to 10 minutes, or until the crust begins to brown. Reduce the temperature to 350° and bake 35 to 40 minutes longer, or until bread is done (golden brown crust on top and bottom, loaf sounds hollow when tapped, loaf shrinks slightly from pan sides). Brush the top crust of the loaves with shortening, then remove the loaves from the pans.

Note: For 1 loaf, cut all the amounts in half.

VARIATIONS:

1. The dough may also be shaped into rolls and baked in muffin pans or on sheet pans (bottoms greased only). Bake at 350° for 20 to 25 minutes, depending on the size of the rolls. Remove from the oven and finish as the bread.

2. For variety, sprinkle caraway seeds on top of the dough before baking.

Rice Flour Yeast Bread‡   Makes 2 loaves

(Wheat-free)

  3 cups rice flour
⅝ cup (10 tablespoons) potato starch
  2 packages active dry yeast
  2 tablespoons granulated sugar
  1 teaspoon salt
  2 tablespoons baking powder
  1 cup dry milk solids
¼ cup instant mashed potatoes
  2 cups very hot water
¼ cup soft butter or margarine
  4 eggs, beaten

Sift the rice flour and potato starch together, then measure 2 cups into a large mixing bowl. Add the yeast, sugar, salt, baking powder, and dry milk and mix thoroughly. Combine the instant mashed potatoes and hot water; whip lightly with a fork. Add the potato mixture and soft butter to the dry ingredients and beat 3 minutes on medium speed. Add the remaining flour and eggs and beat 3 minutes on medium speed; the mixture will be like thick cake batter. Leave the batter in the bowl, cover, and let rise in a warm place for 1 hour. (The batter will rise about 2 inches, depending on the size of the bowl.) Beat just enough to remove the large gas bubbles, then pour the batter into 2 greased 9 x 5-inch loaf pans. Cover and let rise 30 minutes, then bake in a preheated 325° oven for 30 to 35 minutes, until lightly browned.

Note: This bread is especially good when toasted.

Grainless Bread‡ — Makes 1 loaf

(Cereal-free, egg-free)

3 cups Cellu Grainless Mix, sifted
3 teaspoons baking powder
3 tablespoons granulated sugar
1 cup water or milk

Sift the mix into a mixing bowl with the baking powder and sugar. Add the water and stir gently until well mixed. Place the dough in a greased 8 x 3½-inch loaf pan and brush the top with melted butter. Cover the pan loosely with a strip of aluminum foil (which has been pierced in two or three places to release moisture) and place in a preheated 375° oven. Bake at this temperature for 15 minutes, then uncover the pan, reduce the temperature to 350°, and continue baking for 50 minutes more. When done, remove from the pan and place on a wire rack to cool. Store in a plastic bag in the refrigerator.

Orange Nut Bread* — Makes 1 loaf

(Wheat-free, egg-free, milk-free)

2¼ cups ground rolled oats (see note below)
  4 teaspoons baking powder
  ¼ teaspoon baking soda
  ¾ teaspoon salt
  ¾ cup granulated sugar
  ¾ cup chopped nuts
  2 tablespoons melted vegetable shortening or oil
  ¾ cup orange juice
  1 tablespoon grated orange rind

Combine the dry ingredients thoroughly, then add the nuts, shortening, orange juice, and rind. Stir until the dry ingredients are well moistened. Pour into a greased 9 x 5-inch loaf pan and bake in a preheated 350° oven for 60 minutes, or until firm to the touch. To prevent the top of loaf from cracking, cover with aluminum foil during the first 20 minutes of baking.

Note: To grind rolled oats, put them through a food chopper, using the fine cutting blade.

Spoonbread*   Serves 6

(Wheat-free)

3 cups milk
1 cup cornmeal
1½ teaspoons salt
2 tablespoons butter or margarine
4 eggs, separated

Combine the milk, cornmeal, and salt in a saucepan and cook over low heat, stirring constantly, until thickened. Add the butter, then cool. Beat the egg yolks and stir them into the cooled mixture. Beat the egg whites until stiff but not dry, then fold them into the mixture. Pour into a greased 1½-quart casserole and bake in a preheated 400° oven for 35 to 40 minutes, or until set. Serve hot.

Ozark Corn Pone†   Serves 4

(Wheat-free, egg-free, milk-free)

1 cup boiling water
1 cup cornmeal
½ teaspoon salt
2 teaspoons melted vegetable shortening or salad oil

Add the boiling water to the cornmeal and salt; stir to form a stiff dough. Dip your hands in cold water, then mold the mixture into 2 flat ½-inch thick oval cakes. Place on a greased baking sheet and brush with the melted shortening. Bake in a preheated 450° oven for 20 minutes, or until brown and crisp. Cut into pieces and serve as a bread substitute, with maple or fruit syrup.

Muffins, Biscuits, and Crackers

Grainless Muffins‡   Makes 6 muffins

(Cereal-free)

1 cup Cellu Grainless Mix
1 tablespoon granulated sugar
½ cup milk or water
1 egg, beaten

Measure the mix and sugar into a mixing bowl. Add the milk or water and the beaten egg and stir until smooth. Pour into well-oiled muffin tins and bake in a preheated 375° oven for 20 to 25 minutes.

VARIATIONS: **1.** Add ⅓ cup fresh or frozen blueberries, ⅓ cup tart red cherries, or ⅓ cup sliced raw cranberries. **2.** Sprinkle cinnamon and sugar on top of the muffins before baking. **3.** Place 1 tablespoon brown sugar and 1 teaspoon coarse pecan meats in the bottom of the muffin tins and pour the batter on top. **4.** Mix 2 tablespoons Cellu Grainless Mix with 1 tablespoon sugar and grated rind of ⅓ orange. Work into coarse crumbs and sprinkle on top of the muffins before baking.

Cornmeal Muffins*   Makes 10 small muffins

(Wheat-free, egg-free, milk-free)

1 cup cornmeal
½ cup rye flour
⅓ cup rice flour
2 tablespoons baking powder
¾ teaspoon salt
¼ cup granulated sugar
1 cup water
¼ cup melted vegetable shortening

Mix the dry ingredients thoroughly. Add water and shortening and mix well. Fill greased muffin tins about half full. Bake in a preheated 375° oven for 30 minutes, or until very lightly browned and firm to the touch.

Lunch Box Muffins†   Makes 1 dozen muffins

(Wheat-free, egg-free, milk-free)

1 cup oat flour or ground oatmeal
¾ cup rice flour
4 teaspoons baking powder
1 teaspoon salt
1 teaspoon ground cinnamon
½ cup granulated sugar
1¼ cups hot water
½ cup currants or raisins
¼ cup vegetable shortening

Sift together the dry ingredients. Pour hot water over the currants and shortening and add to the dry ingredients. Mix until moistened. Fill greased muffin pans two-thirds full and bake in a preheated 425° oven for 20 minutes.

Cornmeal and Rice Muffiins†

Makes 1 dozen muffins

(Wheat-free, egg-free, milk-free)

⅔ cup cornmeal
1 cup rice flour
4 teaspoons baking powder
½ teaspoon salt
¼ cup granulated sugar
1 cup water
⅓ cup salad oil

Sift together the dry ingredients, then add the water and oil and mix until the dry ingredients are moistened. Fill greased muffin pans two-thirds full and bake in a preheated 375° oven for 20 to 25 minutes.

VARIATION: **Rye Muffins:** Substitute 1 cup rye flour and ½ cup rice flour for the cornmeal and the 1 cup rice flour.

Rye Muffins*

Makes 12 small muffins

(Wheat-free, egg-free, milk-free)

1¼ cups rye flour
½ cup rice flour
4 teaspoons baking powder
¾ teaspoon salt
¼ cup granulated sugar
1 cup water
¼ cup melted vegetable shortening

Combine the dry ingredients thoroughly, then add the water and shortening and mix well. Fill greased muffin tins about half full and bake in a preheated 375° oven for 25 minutes, or until lightly browned.

Rolled Oat Muffins*

Makes 12 medium muffins

(Wheat-free, egg-free, milk-free)

1 cup ground rolled oats (see note below)
¾ cup rice flour
2 tablespoons baking powder
1 teaspoon salt
1 teaspoon cinnamon
¼ cup granulated sugar
½ cup raisins
1¼ cup water
¼ cup melted vegetable shortening

Combine the dry ingredients thoroughly, then add the raisins, water, and shortening and mix well. Fill greased muffin tins about two-thirds full and bake in a preheated 425° oven for 20 minutes, or until lightly browned.

Note: To grind rolled oats, put them through a food chopper, using the fine cutting blade.

Grainless Biscuits‡   Makes 6 biscuits

(Cereal-free, egg-free)

  1 cup Cellu Grainless Mix
  1 tablespoon vegetable shortening
¼ cup milk or water

Combine the mix with the shortening, then add the liquid to make a soft dough. Shape into biscuits and place on a greased baking sheet. Bake in a moderately hot oven (375°) for 25 to 30 minutes.

Rye Biscuits*   Makes 1 dozen 2-inch biscuits

(Wheat-free, egg-free)

1½ cups rye flour
  ½ cup soybean flour
  2 tablespoons granulated sugar
  1 tablespoon baking powder
  1 teaspoon salt
¼ cup vegetable shortening
¾ cup milk, approximately

Thoroughly combine the dry ingredients, then mix in the shortening only until the mixture is crumbly. Add the milk gradually and stir until a soft dough is formed, then place on a floured surface and roll or pat to a thickness of about ½ inch. Cut into 2-inch rounds, place on an ungreased baking sheet, and bake in a preheated 450° oven for 12 minutes, or until very lightly browned.

Oat Biscuits†

Makes 1 dozen biscuits

(Wheat-free, egg-free, milk-free)

1 cup oat flour or ground oatmeal
½ teaspoon salt
3 teaspoons baking powder
1 tablespoon granulated sugar
2 tablespoons vegetable shortening
⅓ cup cold water

Sift together the dry ingredients; cut in the shortening until the mixture is the size of peas. Add the cold water and stir gently to form a soft dough. Knead lightly on a board dusted with oat flour, then roll to a ½-inch thickness. Cut with a 1½-inch round cutter and place on an ungreased baking sheet. Bake in a preheated 450° oven for 15 to 20 minutes.

VARIATIONS: **Coffee Cake:** Add ¼ cup raisins to the dough, spread in an 8-inch pie pan, sprinkle cinnamon and sugar on top, and bake. **Peanut Butter Biscuits:** Substitute 3 tablespoons peanut butter for the shortening. **Rye Biscuits:** Substitute 1 cup rye flour for the oat flour.

Rice Flour Crackers†

Makes 4 dozen crackers

(Wheat-free, egg-free, milk-free)

2 cups rice flour
¼ cup potato starch
1 teaspoon salt
¼ cup sesame seeds
½ cup vegetable shortening
¾ cup water

Sift together the dry ingredients, then add the sesame seeds. Prepare the dough, shape it, and bake as in the recipe for Cornmeal Crackers (page 198).

Cornmeal Crackers†

Makes 4 dozen crackers

(Wheat-free, egg-free, milk-free)

1 cup cornmeal
1 cup rice flour
1 teaspoon salt, more if desired
¼ cup vegetable shortening
½ cup cold water, approximately

Sift together the dry ingredients into a bowl. Cut in the shortening as for pastry, then add the water and stir lightly until the dough holds together. (If too dry, add an additional tablespoon water.)

Divide the dough into 2 parts. Roll each part to a ⅛-inch thickness between 2 sheets of foil. Transfer the foil and dough to a baking sheet. Peel off the top sheet of foil and cut the dough into squares. Sprinkle with salt, if desired. Bake in a preheated 325° oven for 15 minutes, or until lightly browned.

VARIATION: **Rye Crackers:** Substitute 2 cups rye flour for the cornmeal and rice flour.

Oatmeal Crackers†   Makes 4 dozen crackers

(Wheat-free, egg-free, milk-free)

4 cups oatmeal
½ cup salad oil
2 tablespoons granulated sugar
1 teaspoon salt
¾ cup lukewarm water

Thoroughly combine the oatmeal and salad oil. Mix in the sugar and salt, then add the water and mix well. (The dough will be slightly sticky.) For shaping and baking, follow instructions in the preceding recipe for Cornmeal Crackers.

Rye Crackers*   Makes about 75 crackers

(Wheat-free, egg-free)

1¾ cups rye flour
1 cup rice flour
1½ teaspoons salt
1 teaspoon baking soda
½ cup butter or margarine
1 cup buttermilk

Combine the dry ingredients thoroughly, then mix in the butter only until the mixture is crumbly. Add the buttermilk and mix well.

Place the dough on a well-floured surface and roll very thin. Cut into 3 x 1½-inch strips and place, with sides touching, on a baking sheet. Bake in a preheated 375° oven for 18 minutes, or until lightly browned.

Note: Sprinkle the tops of the crackers with coarse salt before baking, if desired.

Grainless Wafers‡   Makes about 2 dozen wafers

(Cereal-free, egg-free)

½ cup Cellu Grainless Mix
¼ cup Cellu Soy Grits
 1 tablespoon granulated sugar
¼ cup Cellu Evaporated Goat Milk

Place all the ingredients in a mixing bowl and stir until the dough forms into a ball. Work the dough in your hands until it becomes elastic, then roll or pat into a thin sheet and place in a large pie plate or flat cake tin. Bake in a preheated 325° oven for 30 to 35 minutes. To eat, break into pieces.

Pancakes, Waffles, and Dumplings

Buckwheat Pancakes†   Makes 16 pancakes

(Wheat-free, egg-free, milk-free)

 1 package active dry yeast
 1 tablespoon brown sugar
 2 cups buckwheat flour
½ cup cornmeal
 1 teaspoon salt
2½ cups hot water
 1 teaspoon baking soda
 1 teaspoon warm water
 2 tablespoons salad oil

Thoroughly combine all dry ingredients except the baking soda in a mixer bowl. Add the hot water and beat for 2 minutes on medium speed. Cover and allow to rise overnight in a warm place.

In the morning, stir the mixture well, then add the baking soda dissolved in the warm water and oil; mix again. Pour onto a hot greased griddle and cook until golden brown on both sides. Serve with syrup.

Wheatless Waffles*   Makes 16 seven-inch waffles

(Wheat-free)

1½ cups rice flour
 1 tablespoon baking powder
 1 teaspoon salt
1½ cups milk
 2 eggs, separated
 3 tablespoons melted shortening or oil

Combine the dry ingredients thoroughly, then beat in the milk, egg yolks, and shortening. Stiffly beat the egg whites and fold in. Bake in a hot waffle iron.

Grainless Waffles‡   Makes 1 waffle

(Cereal-free)

1 egg, separated
2 tablespoons milk or water
¼ cup Cellu Grainless Mix
1 teaspoon granulated sugar (optional)

Add the egg yolk to the milk and beat until blended. Add the liquid to the mix and stir until smooth. Beat the egg white until stiff and fold it into the flour mixture. Pour onto a hot waffle iron and bake until brown.

Note: When made with water, add 1 teaspoon sugar to the batter to facilitate browning.

Rice Flour Waffles or Pancakes†   Makes 12 waffles or 8 pancakes

(Wheat-free, egg-free, milk-free)

2 cups rice flour
4 teaspoons baking powder
½ teaspoon salt
1 tablespoon granulated sugar
2 cups water
3 tablespoons salad oil

Sift together the dry ingredients, then add the water and oil gradually, stirring the mixture constantly until smooth. Pour onto a heated waffle iron or griddle and bake until golden brown. Serve with syrup.

Dumplings‡   Makes about 1 dozen dumplings

(Cereal-free)

1 tablespoon beaten egg
½ cup Cellu Grainless Mix
¾ tablespoon Cellu Evaporated Goat Milk

Combine all the ingredients in a small mixing bowl and work to a smooth dough. Drop the dough into a small steamer pan, cover, and cook over boiling water for 15 to 18 minutes. Serve with meat stews or creamed meats.

Note: These may also be dropped (using ½ teaspoon portions) into boiling broth and then served in it.

VARIATION: **Fruit Dumplings:** To the ingredients listed above, add 1 tablespoon sugar and stir to a smooth mixture. Drop by spoonfuls into a pan of boiling fruit (use one-pound can of either tart red cherries, prune plums, or blueberries). Cover and let cook slowly for about 15 minutes.

Note: The dumplings, which make a good dessert, may also be placed in the oven to bake.

Stuffings and Dressings

Cornbread Stuffing†   Enough to stuff a 12-pound turkey

(Wheat-free, egg-free, milk-free)

   6 cups cornbread crumbs (choose a recipe tolerated)
1½ cups chopped onion or ⅓ cup instant chopped onion
1½ cups chopped celery and celery leaves
   ½ cup vegetable shortening or milk-free margarine
   1 tablespoon salt
   ½ teaspoon pepper
   1 tablespoon poultry seasoning
   1 cup water or turkey or chicken broth

Put the cornbread crumbs on a baking sheet and dry out in a 200° oven for 30 minutes. Sauté the onion and celery in the shortening. Add the seasonings and liquid, pour over the crumbs, and mix until the crumbs are moistened. Stuff the turkey and bake immediately, or bake separately in a greased 2-quart casserole.

VARIATIONS: **Bacon Dressing:** ¼ pound crumbled, crisp-fried bacon may be added. **Mushroom Dressing:** 1 pint sliced fresh mushrooms may be sautéed with the onions and celery or 1 two-and-one-half-ounce can mushroom pieces may be added. **Oyster Dressing:** 1 pint oysters may be added to the sautéed onions and celery and heated just until the edges curl. **Sausage Dressing:** ½ pound thoroughly fried sausage may be added. **Water Chestnut Dressing:** ½ cup thinly sliced chestnuts may be added.

Oatmeal Dressing†   Enough to stuff a 4-pound chicken

(Wheat-free, egg-free, milk-free)

⅓ cup butter-flavored oil
⅓ cup chopped onion or 2 tablespoons instant chopped onion
 1 cup oatmeal

Combine the ingredients, stuff a chicken, and bake.

Rice Almond Dressing†   Enough to stuff a 4-pound chicken

(Wheat-free, egg-free, milk-free)

¼ cup salad oil
¼ cup minced onion or 1 tablespoon instant chopped onion
½ cup raw rice
 1 cup chicken broth
 1 teaspoon salt
½ cup chopped almonds (if tolerated)

Heat the oil in a large skillet. Add the onion and rice and sauté over low heat, stirring frequently, until the rice is golden. Stir in the broth and salt, cover and simmer for 15 minutes, stirring occasionally, or until the rice is tender. Remove from the heat and stir in the almonds. Stuff a chicken and bake, or bake in a casserole for 30 minutes.

Tomato Dressing†   Enough to stuff a 4-pound chicken

(Wheat-free, egg-free, milk-free)

 2 tablespoons salad oil
¼ cup chopped onion or 1 tablespoon instant chopped onion
½ cup raw rice
 1 one-pound can tomatoes
 1 teaspoon salt
¼ teaspoon pepper
¼ teaspoon chili powder

Heat the oil in a skillet and sauté the onion and rice, stirring frequently, until the rice is golden. Stir in the remaining ingredients, bring to a boil, cover, and simmer for 15 minutes, or until liquid has been absorbed and the rice is tender. Stuff a chicken and bake, or bake in a casserole for 30 minutes.

Pie Crusts and Pies

Grainless Pie Crust‡

Makes 2 small pie shells

(Cereal-free, egg-free, milk-free)

½ cup Cellu Grainless Mix
1 tablespoon vegetable shortening
1½ tablespoons warm water

Combine all the ingredients in a mixing bowl and work for a short while with the hands to form a smooth ball. Roll or press into shape in two small 4½-inch pie tins. Prick well and bake in a preheated 325° oven for about 15 minutes.

Corn Flake or Rice Flake Piecrust*

Makes 1 nine-inch pie shell

(Wheat-free, egg-free)

1 cup crushed corn or rice flakes
¼ cup granulated sugar
⅓ cup melted butter or margarine

Thoroughly combine all the ingredients and press into a 9-inch pie pan. Bake for 5 to 8 minutes in a preheated 375° oven, then cool before filling.

Barley Pie Crust†

Makes 1 nine-inch pie shell

(Wheat-free, egg-free, milk-free)

1½ cups barley flour
1 teaspoon granulated sugar
½ teaspoon salt
⅓ cup vegetable shortening
¼ cup cold water

Sift together the dry ingredients, then cut in the shortening until the mixture is the size of peas. Add the cold water, a little at a time, until a ball is formed. Place the dough between 2 sheets of foil and roll to a thickness of ⅛ inch. Transfer the foil and dough to a pie pan. Fit into the pan, then peel off the top foil; trim the edges of the dough and bottom foil to fit the pan. Prick the dough with fork and bake in a preheated 350° oven for 15 minutes, or until brown. (Browning is very important for flavor.)

VARIATIONS: **Rice Crust:** Substitute ¾ cup rice flour for the barley flour.

This crust can be pressed into the pan instead of rolling. **Rye Crust:** Substitute 1½ cups rye flour for the barley flour.

Crumb Crust†　　　　　　　　　　　Makes 1 nine-inch pie shell

(Wheat-free, egg-free, milk-free)

1 cup crushed rice cereal
¼ cup granulated sugar
⅓ cup melted milk-free margarine or vegetable shortening

Combine the cereal crumbs, sugar, and melted shortening and press firmly into the bottom and sides of a 9-inch pie pan. Bake in a preheated 375° oven for 8 minutes, or until lightly browned.
Note: Instead of baking the crust, it may be refrigerated for 1 hour and then filled.

VARIATIONS: Crushed corn cereal or oatmeal may be used in place of rice cereal. The oatmeal crust must be baked.

Coconut Crust†　　　　　　　　　　Makes 1 nine-inch pie shell

(Wheat-free, egg-free, milk-free)

¼ cup melted milk-free margarine or shortening
2 cups flake-type coconut

Combine the melted shortening and coconut. Press evenly into an ungreased 9-inch pie pan and bake in a preheated 300° oven for 30 to 35 minutes, or until lightly browned.
Note: This and all crusts may be filled with fruited gelatin or fruits thickened with tapioca or cornstarch.

Apricot Cream Pie†　　　　　　　　　Makes 1 nine-inch pie

(Wheat-free, egg-free, milk-free)

1 envelope unflavored gelatin
¼ cup cold water
1 cup apricot pulp, strained or blended
½ cup apricot juice
2 tablespoons lemon juice
⅓ cup granulated sugar
¼ teaspoon salt
1 cup whipped nondairy topping
1 baked nine-inch pie shell

Soften the gelatin in the cold water. Heat together the apricot pulp and juice, lemon juice, sugar, and salt. Add the soaked gelatin and stir until dissolved.

Chill until partially set, then whip until light and fluffy. Fold in the whipped topping and pour into a baked pie crust; chill until set.

Note: The pie may be garnished with additional whipped topping.

Lemon Pie†   Makes 1 nine-inch pie

(Wheat-free, egg-free, milk-free)

1 cup granulated sugar
¼ cup cornstarch or ½ cup rice flour
½ teaspoon salt
1 cup water
2 tablespoons grated lemon rind
½ cup lemon juice
2 tablespoons milk-free margarine
1 baked 9-inch pie shell

Combine the sugar, cornstarch or rice flour, and salt together in a saucepan. Stir the water in gradually and cook over medium heat, stirring constantly, until the mixture thickens and boils. When the mixture is clear, add the lemon rind, juice, and margarine. Remove from heat and chill.

When ready to serve, spoon into the baked pie crust. Chill until serving time.

Note: This may be garnished with whipped nondairy topping.

Pumpkin Pie†   Makes 1 nine-inch pie

(Wheat-free, egg-free, milk-free)

2 cups canned pumpkin
⅔ cup plus ½ cup brown sugar, firmly packed
1½ cups water
6 tablespoons cornstarch
1 tablespoon pumpkin spice (or spices tolerated)
½ teaspoon salt
1 unbaked nine-inch barley, rice, or rye pie shell
¼ cup coconut
¼ cup chopped pecans (if tolerated)

Combine all the ingredients except the ½ cup sugar, the coconut, and pecans in a saucepan. Cook over low heat until the mixture begins to thicken, stirring constantly. Pour into the pie crust and bake in a preheated 375° oven for 30 minutes. Combine the remaining brown sugar, coconut, and pecans and sprinkle on top of the pie. Bake for 5 minutes more.

Raspberry Minute Pie†   Makes 1 nine-inch pie

(Wheat-free, egg-free, milk-free)

1 three-ounce package raspberry gelatin
1 cup boiling water
1 ten-ounce package frozen raspberries
  Whipped nondairy topping (optional)
1 nine-inch crumb crust

Dissolve the gelatin in the boiling water. Add the raspberries and stir, breaking up the frozen berries with a fork.

As the berries defrost, the gelatin will thicken. When partially set, pour into the crumb crust. Refrigerate until completely set. Serve with nondairy dessert topping if desired.

VARIATION: Substitute strawberry gelatin for the raspberry and frozen strawberries for raspberries.

Puddings, Frozen Desserts, and Dessert Sauces

Fig-Nut Pudding*   Serves 6

(Wheat-free, milk-free)

  2 eggs
¾ cup granulated sugar
  3 tablespoons rice flour
  1 teaspoon baking powder
¼ teaspoon salt
½ teaspoon ground cinnamon
  1 cup chopped dried figs
  1 cup chopped nuts

Beat the eggs until thick and light in color. Add the sugar to the eggs gradually, beating constantly. Combine the dry ingredients and stir into the egg mixture, then add the figs and nuts and beat thoroughly. Pour into a greased 8 x 2-inch pan and bake in a preheated 300° oven for 40 minutes, or until the mixture is firm to the touch.

Lemon Delight†   Serves 9

(Wheat-free, egg-free, milk-free)

1¾ cups water
  1 three-ounce package lemon gelatin
  3 tablespoons lemon juice
  ½ teaspoon shredded lemon peel
  1 teaspoon vanilla extract
  ⅓ cup confectioners' sugar
1½ cups rice cereal, crushed to ⅓ cup
  2 tablespoons chopped, toasted almonds
  3 tablespoons soft milk-free margarine
  1 cup whipped non-dairy topping

Heat 1 cup of the water to boiling. Dissolve the gelatin in it, then add the remaining ¾ cup water, lemon juice, peel, vanilla, and confectioners' sugar. Chill until very thick.

Combine the rice cereal crumbs, almonds, and margarine and press a heaping teaspoonful into the bottom of each of 9 six-ounce molds. Whip the gelatin mixture until fluffy and thick; fold in whipped topping and pour into the molds. Sprinkle the remaining crumbs on top and chill 3 to 4 hours. To serve, invert on plates.

Note: These are good when frozen.

Apricot Sherbet†   Makes 1½ quarts

(Wheat-free, egg-free, milk-free)

  1 envelope unflavored gelatin
  ½ cup cold water
  2 twelve-ounce cans apricot nectar
  ¾ cup light corn syrup
  ¼ cup lemon juice
  ⅛ teaspoon salt

Put the water in a saucepan and sprinkle on the gelatin. Place over low heat and stir constantly until the gelatin is dissolved. Stir in the remaining ingredients and pour into 2 refrigerator trays. Freeze until firm (about 1 hour), then beat in a chilled bowl until light and creamy. Return to the refrigerator trays and freeze until firm (2 or 3 hours).

Orange Ice†   Makes 2 quarts

(Wheat-free, egg-free, milk-free)

    2 cups granulated sugar
    1 quart water
    2 cups orange juice
    ¼ cup lemon juice
      Grated rind of 2 oranges

Boil the sugar and water for 5 minutes. Add the fruit juices and grated rind and cool, strain, and freeze.

VARIATION: 1. Apricot Sherbet (page 208) and Orange Ice (above) may be mixed according to directions and then frozen until mushy in sectioned ice trays. Insert popsicle sticks. 2. Flavored beverage powders may be mixed according to package directions and then frozen in sectional ice trays. 3. Any other fruit juice or tomato juice may also be substituted in the above recipe.

Fruit Sauce†   Makes 1 cup sauce

(Wheat-free, egg-free, milk-free)

    1 cup fruit juice (apricot, cherry, peach, grape, or pineapple)
    2 tablespoons granulated sugar
    1 tablespoon cornstarch or 2 tablespoons rice flour
    2 tablespoons cold water

Heat the juice and sugar to boiling. Mix the cornstarch or rice flour and cold water to a smooth paste, then add to the hot juice, stirring constantly. Cook slowly until thick and clear.
    Note: This sauce may be served with fruit pudding, boiled rice, desserts, or allowed cereals.

Cakes

Fudge Cake†   Serves 12

(Wheat-free, egg-free, milk-free)

  1 cup soybean flour
½ cup potato starch
¼ cup cocoa
½ teaspoon salt
  2 teaspoons baking powder
  1 teaspoon baking soda
  1 teaspoon black walnut extract or vanilla extract
  1 tablespoon vinegar
½ cup salad oil
  1 cup cold water

Sift together all the dry ingredients, then add the liquids and beat at
medium speed for 3 minutes, until the batter is very smooth. Pour into
a greased 9 x 9 x 2-inch pan and bake in a preheated 300° oven for 40
minutes. Do not remove the cake from pan, but frost immediately with the
following icing:

Fudge Icing   Makes about 1 cup

(Wheat-free, egg-free, milk-free)

  1 cup granulated sugar
¼ cup cocoa (see note below)
½ cup vegetable shortening or milk-free margarine
¼ cup strong, hot coffee

Put all the ingredients in a heavy saucepan. Bring to a boil and boil for
1 minute. Pour over the cake immediately.
  Note: Carob powder may be substituted if chocolate is not tolerated.

Nougat Gold Cake†   Serves 16

(Wheat-free, egg-free, milk-free)

  1 one-pound can crushed pineapple, undrained
  1 cup brown sugar, firmly packed
½ cup vegetable shortening or milk-free margarine

1 cup water
1½ cups raisins
½ cup chopped dates
3 tablespoons instant sweet potatoes
1 tablespoon pumpkin pie spice (or spices tolerated)
1¼ cups rice flour
½ cup soybean flour
1 teaspoon baking soda
2 teaspoons baking powder
½ cup chopped nuts (if tolerated)

Combine the pineapple, sugar, shortening, water, raisins, dates, sweet potatoes, and spice in a 3-quart saucepan. Bring to a boil, then simmer, uncovered, for 5 minutes. Add the rice flour and stir well. Cool.

Sift together the soybean flour, baking soda, and baking powder. Add to the cooked mixture and combine thoroughly. Add the nuts, pour into a greased 8 x 11-inch baking pan, and bake for 1 hour in a preheated 300° oven. When cool, dust with confectioners' sugar.

Note: This is a very moist cake.

Popcorn Confetti Cake†   Serves 16

(Wheat-free, egg-free, milk-free)

1 cup granulated sugar
1 cup white corn syrup
½ cup water
2 tablespoons milk-free margarine
Few drops food coloring (optional)
4 quarts popped corn
2 cups small colored gumdrops

Combine the sugar, corn syrup, water, and milk-free margarine in a saucepan. Cook to 240°, or until a little dropped into cold water forms a soft ball. Add coloring, if desired.

Pour the syrup over the popped corn combined with the gumdrops and mix well. Press the mixture into a well-greased 10-inch tube pan and unmold immediately. To serve, slice with a sharp knife.

Note: Decorated with candles, this makes a novel birthday cake. It can be wrapped and frozen.

Pineapple Cake‡

Serves 6

(Cereal-free, milk-free)

¾ cup drained, crushed pineapple
2 eggs, separated
½ cup granulated sugar
¼ teaspoon salt
1½ cups Cellu Grainless Mix
3 tablespoons pineapple juice

Place the drained pineapple in a mixing bowl and add the egg yolks, sugar, and salt. Combine thoroughly, then gradually stir in the mix and the pineapple juice. Beat the egg whites stiff and fold in. Pour into a 7 x 7-inch baking pan and bake in a preheated 350° oven for 35 to 40 minutes.

Pineapple Upside-Down Cake*

Serves 9

(Wheat-free, egg-free, milk-free)

¼ cup plus ⅓ cup vegetable shortening
½ cup plus ⅔ cup brown sugar, packed
6 slices canned pineapple, drained and liquid reserved
1 cup rye flour
¾ cup rice flour
½ teaspoon salt
4 teaspoons baking powder

Melt the ¼ cup shortening with the ½ cup brown sugar in an 8 x 8 x 2-inch baking pan in the oven. Arrange the pineapple slices in the sugar mixture. Beat the ⅓ cup shortening and the ⅔ cup brown sugar together until very creamy and fluffy. Combine the dry ingredients thoroughly, then add, alternately with the pineapple liquid (combined with enough water to make 1 cup), to the creamy mixture. Beat well after each addition.

Pour the batter over the pineapple and bake in a preheated 375° oven for 45 minutes, or until the cake begins to leave the sides of the pan. Invert, in the pan, on a plate. The cake will come out of pan in a few minutes. Serve while still warm.

Date Cake*

Serves 9

(Wheat-free, milk-free)

1 cup boiling water
1 cup chopped dates
1 cup granulated sugar
½ cup vegetable shortening
1 egg, beaten
1 teaspoon vanilla extract
1½ cups rice flour
¾ cup soybean flour
4 teaspoons baking powder
¼ teaspoon salt
¼ teaspoon grated nutmeg

Pour the boiling water over the dates and cool to lukewarm. Adding the sugar gradually, beat the shortening and sugar together until the mixture is very creamy. Beat well after each addition. Add the egg and vanilla and beat well.

Combine the dry ingredients thoroughly and add, alternately with the dates, to the shortening mixture. Beat well after each addition. Pour into a greased 8 x 8 x 2-inch baking pan and bake in a preheated 350° oven for 50 minutes, or until the cake begins to leave the sides of the pan. The cake may be served warm or cold.

Note: Top the cooled cake with a creamy frosting, made by blending together 1¼ cups confectioners' sugar, 3 tablespoons shortening, ½ teaspoon desired flavoring, and enough water or fruit juice for a good spreading consistency.

Spice Cake*

Serves 9

(Wheat-free, egg-free, milk-free)

1¼ cups boiling water
1 cup raisins
1 cup brown sugar, packed
⅓ cup vegetable shortening
1 teaspoon vanilla extract
1 cup rye flour
½ teaspoon salt
1 teaspoon grated nutmeg
1 teaspoon ground cinnamon
4 teaspoons baking powder
1 cup cornmeal

Pour the boiling water over the raisins and cool to lukewarm. Adding the sugar gradually, beat the shortening, brown sugar, and vanilla together until very creamy and fluffy. Combine the dry ingredients thoroughly, then add, alternately with the raisins, to the shortening mixture. Beat well after each addition.

Pour into a greased 8 x 8 x 2-inch baking pan and bake in a preheated 375° oven for 45 minutes, or until the cake begins to leave the sides of the pan. Serve warm, if desired.

Chiffon Cake*   Serves 9

(Wheat-free, milk-free)

¾ cup rice flour
¾ cup granulated sugar
1½ teaspoons baking powder
½ teaspoon salt
¼ cup vegetable oil
3 eggs, separated
¼ cup water
1 tablespoon lemon juice
1 teaspoon grated lemon rind
¼ teaspoon cream of tartar

Combine the dry ingredients thoroughly, then add the oil, egg yolks, water, lemon juice, and rind and beat until very smooth. Beat the egg whites with the cream of tartar until stiff but not dry and fold into egg-yolk mixture. Pour into an ungreased 8 x 8 x 2-inch baking pan and bake in a preheated 350° oven for 35 minutes, or until firm to the touch. Invert, in the pan, on a rack to cool.

Molasses Sheet Bread‡   Serves 6

(Cereal-free, egg-free, milk-free)

1 cup Cellu Grainless Mix
½ teaspoon ground ginger
¼ teaspoon baking soda
¼ cup brown sugar
¼ cup cane molasses
6 tablespoons water

Mix the dry ingredients, then combine with the molasses and water. Pour into a greased pie tin or small square (7 x 7-inch) baking pan and bake in a moderate oven (350°) for 30 to 40 minutes.

Note: If allowed, raisins may be added.

Cookies and Candy

Oatmeal Lace Cookies*

Makes 5 dozen medium cookies

(Wheat-free, egg-free, milk-free)

1 cup brown sugar, packed
1 cup granulated sugar
1 cup vegetable shortening
1 teaspoon vanilla extract
1 cup rice flour
1 teaspoon salt
4 teaspoons baking powder
¾ cup water
3 cups quick-cooking rolled oats
½ cup chopped nuts

Adding the sugars gradually, beat the shortening, sugars, and vanilla together until fluffy. Thoroughly combine the flour, salt, and baking powder, then add, alternately with the water, to the shortening mixture. Add the rolled oats and nuts and mix well. Chill overnight.

The following day, drop the batter by teaspoonfuls onto lightly greased baking sheets. Bake in a preheated 350° oven for 10 minutes, or until lightly browned.

Molasses Drop Cookies*

Makes 4 dozen cookies

(Wheat-free, egg-free, milk-free)

½ cup vegetable shortening
½ cup brown sugar, packed
½ cup molasses
1¾ cups rye flour
1 teaspoon ground ginger
1 teaspoon ground cinnamon
¼ teaspoon ground cloves
¼ teaspoon salt
1½ teaspoons baking powder
¼ teaspoon baking soda
⅓ cup water
½ teaspoon vinegar

Beat the shortening and brown sugar together until very creamy and fluffy, then beat in the molasses. Combine the dry ingredients thoroughly and add, alternately with the water and vinegar, to the shortening mixture, beating well after each addition. Chill thoroughly.

Drop the batter by teaspoonfuls onto lightly greased baking sheets and bake in a preheated 350° oven for 8 to 10 minutes, or until lightly browned and set.

Applesauce Cookies†   Makes 2 dozen cookies

(Wheat-free, egg-free, milk-free)

¼ cup salad oil
½ cup brown sugar, firmly packed
¼ cup granulated sugar
½ cup thick applesauce
1 teaspoon vanilla extract
1 cup potato starch
⅛ teaspoon baking soda
2 teaspoons baking powder
¼ cup chopped nuts (if tolerated)

Combine the oil and the sugars, then add the applesauce and vanilla. Sift together the dry ingredients and stir into the sugar mixture; add the nuts. Drop by teaspoonfuls on a greased cookie sheet and bake in a preheated 350° oven for 12 minutes, or until lightly browned.

Rice Cookies†   Makes 2 dozen cookies

(Wheat-free, egg-free, milk-free)

1¼ cups rice flour
¼ teaspoon baking soda
1 teaspoon baking powder
¼ teaspoon salt
½ cup granulated sugar
¼ cup salad oil
2 teaspoons vanilla extract
1 teaspoon butter flavoring
¼ cup water

Sift together all the dry ingredients, then add the salad oil, vanilla, butter flavoring, and water and mix well. Drop the batter by teaspoonfuls on a greased baking sheet and bake in a preheated 350° oven for 15 minutes, or until lightly browned.

Grainless Coconut Cookies‡   Makes about 2 dozen cookies

(Cereal-free, egg-free)

1 cup Cellu Grainless Mix
⅓ cup granulated sugar
⅓ cup shredded coconut
⅓ cup Cellu Evaporated Goat Milk
½ teaspoon vanilla extract

Place all the ingredients in a bowl and stir until dough is of a soft consistency and well mixed. Form into small balls and place on a cookie sheet. Bake in a preheated 350° oven for 12 to 15 minutes.

Coconut Cookies†   Makes 2 dozen cookies

(Wheat-free, egg-free, milk-free)

⅓ cup brown sugar, firmly packed
¼ cup salad oil
3 tablespoons flake-type coconut
1 teaspoon vanilla extract
1 teaspoon butter flavoring
1 cup rice flour
2 teaspoons baking powder
¼ teaspoon salt
¼ cup cold water

Combine the sugar and oil, then add the coconut and flavorings. Sift together the rice flour, baking powder, and salt. Add, alternately with the water, to the creamed mixture. Stir into a smooth dough, then form into a roll and wrap in foil. Chill in the refrigerator.

Cut the dough into ¼-inch slices. Place on a greased baking sheet and bake in a preheated 375° oven for 20 minutes, or until lightly browned.

Jack and Jill Cookies†   Makes 3 dozen cookies

(Wheat-free, egg-free, milk-free)

¼ cup salad oil
½ cup granulated sugar
2 cups dry baby-food rice cereal
2 teaspoons baking powder
1 four-and-three-quarter-ounce jar strained peaches
1 teaspoon almond extract

Combine all the ingredients and stir lightly until the mixture holds together. Form into 1-inch balls, press thin on a greased baking sheet, and bake in a preheated 325° oven for 15 minutes.

Note: These cookies have crisp edges and a chewy center.

Apricot Cookies‡   Makes about 2 dozen cookies

(Cereal-free, egg-free)

  1 cup Cellu Grainless Mix
  2 tablespoons vegetable shortening
  3 tablespoons brown sugar
  3 tablespoons granulated sugar
½ teaspoon ground cinnamon or vanilla extract
⅓ cup fruit juice (apricot, peach, or orange)
    Dried apricots, cut up.

Combine the mix and shortening in a bowl, then add the sugars and cinnamon. Add the fruit juice and stir to a smooth dough. Add the dried apricots, then drop onto a cookie sheet and bake in a preheated 350° oven for 12 to 15 minutes.

Fig Bars*   Makes 40 bars

(Wheat-free, milk-free)

  1 cup chopped dried figs
  1 cup chopped nuts
  1 cup sifted confectioners' sugar, more if desired
  2 eggs, beaten
¼ cup rice flour
½ teaspoon salt
  1 tablespoon melted vegetable shortening or oil
  1 tablespoon lemon juice

Thoroughly combine the figs, nuts, sugar, and eggs. Combine the flour and salt and stir into the fig mixture. Add the shortening and lemon juice and beat well.

Spread the mixture in a greased 8 x 8 x 2-inch baking pan and bake in a preheated 325° oven for 40 minutes, or until lightly browned. Cool, then cut into ¾ x 2-inch bars. Roll the bars in additional confectioners' sugar, if desired.

Raisin Nut Bars†   Makes 2 dozen bars

(Wheat-free, egg-free, milk-free)

 1 cup brown sugar, firmly packed
 1 cup water
 2 tablespoons salad oil
 1 teaspoon ground cinnamon
 1 teaspoon grated nutmeg
 ¼ teaspoon ground cloves
 ¼ teaspoon salt
 1 cup raisins
24 rye wafers rolled into crumbs
 ½ teaspoon baking soda
 ½ cup chopped nuts (if tolerated)
 1 tablespoon warm water
 1 teaspoon lemon juice

Combine the sugar, water, oil, cinnamon, nutmeg, cloves, salt, and raisins and boil together for 5 minutes, stirring frequently. Remove from the heat and stir in the rye wafers, baking soda, and nuts. Pour into a greased 8 x 8 x 2-inch pan and bake in a preheated 350° oven for 30 minutes. Make a glaze by combining the 1 tablespoon warm water, lemon juice, and confectioners' sugar. Spread on the warm cake, then cool and cut into bars.

Chinese Chews†   Makes 16 squares

(Wheat-free, egg-free, milk-free)

 1 cup chopped dried dates, figs, prunes, or apricots
 ¼ cup granulated sugar
 6 tablespoons water
 2 tablespoons lemon juice
 2 cups oatmeal
 ½ teaspoon baking soda
 ½ cup brown sugar, firmly packed
 ½ cup vegetable shortening or milk-free margarine
 2 tablespoons water

Combine the fruit, sugar, and ¼ cup water and cook until smooth; add the lemon juice and cool.

   Combine the oatmeal, baking soda, and brown sugar; cut in the shortening to make crumbs. Set aside one-third of the crumb mixture for the topping. Add the remaining 2 tablespoons water to the remainder and pack into a greased 8 x 8 x 2-inch pan. Spread the fruit filling over and sprinkle the top with crumbs. Bake in a preheated 350° oven for 30 minutes. To serve, cut into squares.

Scotch Toffee†
Makes 32 bars

(Wheat-free, egg-free, milk-free)

½ cup vegetable shortening or milk-free margarine
½ cup brown sugar, firmly packed
¼ cup dark corn syrup
½ teaspoon salt
1 teaspoon vanilla extract
2 cups oatmeal
1 six-ounce package butterscotch chips
½ cup chopped nuts (if tolerated)

Melt the shortening, then add all the other ingredients except the butterscotch chips and nuts and mix well. Pat evenly into a greased 8 x 8 x 2-inch pan and bake for 7 minutes in a preheated 400° oven, or until slightly brown around the edges. (The mixture will be soft and bubbling but will harden as it cools.) Melt the butterscotch chips over hot water. Spread over the top, then sprinkle with nuts. Cut into bars when set.

Cinnamon Munch†
Makes 2 cups

(Wheat-free, egg-free, milk-free)

¼ cup granulated sugar
1 teaspoon ground cinnamon
3 tablespoons milk-free margarine
2 cups bite-sized shredded rice biscuits

Combine the sugar and cinnamon and set aside. Melt the margarine in a skillet over low heat, then add the cereal and stir gently until each piece is coated. Sprinkle the sugar-cinnamon mixture over the cereal. Continue to heat, stirring gently until the biscuits are evenly covered. Turn into a bowl and serve as snacks, either warm or cold.

Marshmallow Crispies†
Makes 2 dozen bars

(Wheat-free, egg-free, milk-free)

2 tablespoons milk-free margarine
1 cup marshmallow creme or 2 cups miniature marshmallows
3 cups crisp rice cereal

Melt the margarine in a saucepan over low heat, then add the marshmallow creme and heat until melted (5 minutes). Remove from the heat and stir in the cereal. Pack firmly into an 8 x 8-inch pan greased with milk-free margarine. Let stand until firm, then cut into bars.

Butterscotch Jumbles†

Makes 2 dozen jumbles

(Wheat-free, egg-free, milk-free)

  1 six-ounce package butterscotch chips
½ cup corn syrup
1¾ cups crisp rice cereal

Melt chips over boiling water and blend with the syrup. Remove from the heat, but leave over hot water. Add the cereal; mix gently until each piece is covered with the butterscotch mixture. Drop by heaping teaspoonfuls on waxed paper. Let stand until firm.

VARIATION: Chocolate chips and crisp corn cereal may be substituted for the butterscotch and rice cereal.

Marshmallow Pops†

Makes 15 pops

(Wheat-free, egg-free, milk-free)

  1 six-ounce package butterscotch chips
16 large marshmallows
1½ cups crushed corn or rice cereal

Melt the butterscotch chips over hot water. Insert a popsicle stick in center of each marshmallow and dip the marshmallow into the melted chips. Press the crushed cereal into each coated marshmallow until completely covered, then place on a waxed paper-lined tray. Chill at least 30 minutes, until the coating is firm.

Peanut Butter Balls†

Makes 2 dozen balls

(Wheat-free, egg-free, milk-free)

½ cup peanut butter
 2 tablespoons lemon juice
 1 cup chopped dates
½ cup sifted confectioners' sugar

Mix the peanut butter, lemon juice, and dates and form into ½-inch balls. Roll the balls in confectioners' sugar.

Turkish Bars†   Makes 4 dozen bars

(Wheat-free, egg-free, milk-free)

   3 envelopes unflavored gelatin
   3 cups granulated sugar, approximately
 ¼ teaspoon salt
1¾ cups cold water
   1 teaspoon vanilla extract
   1 tablespoon lemon juice
   Few drops yellow or green food coloring

Combine the gelatin, 2 cups of the sugar, and salt in a 2-quart saucepan. Add the water and bring to a boil. Boil, stirring occasionally, until a candy thermometer reads 222°F. (about 10 minutes). Remove from the heat and add the vanilla, lemon juice, and food coloring. Pour into an 8 x 8 x 2-inch square pan that has been rinsed in cold water. Let stand at room temperature until very firm (12 hours), then cut into bars with a wet knife. Remove from the pan and roll in the remaining granulated sugar.

ALLERGY-FREE RECIPES:
A SELECTED BIBLIOGRAPHY

General:

Allergy Diets. Ralston Purina Company, Checkerboard Square, St. Louis, Mo. 63199.

Allergy Recipes. The American Dietetic Association, 620 North Michigan Avenue, Chicago, Ill. 60611. Price: $.50.

Allergy Recipes from the Blue Flame Kitchen. Metropolitan Utilities District, 1723 Harney Street, Omaha, Neb. 68102. Price: $.50.

Baking for People with Food Allergies. Superintendent of Documents, U.S. Government Printing Office, Washington, D.C. 20402.

Cooper's Nutrition in Health & Disease Book. H. S. Mitchell, H. J. Rynbergen, L. Anderson, and M. V. Dibble. Philadelphia: J. B. Lippincott, 1968.

Good Recipes to Brighten the Allergy Diet. Best Foods, A Division of CPC International, Inc., Dept. AB, Englewood Cliffs, N.J. 07632. Free.

125 Great Recipes for Allergy Diets. Good Housekeeping Institute, 959 Fifth Avenue, New York, N.Y. 10019. Price: $.50. A collection of egg-, gluten-, milk-, and/or wheat-free recipes.

Recipes Using Barley Flour and *Recipes Using Soybean Flour.* The Chicago Dietetic Supply House, Incorporated, 1750 West Van Buren Street, Chicago, Ill. 60612. This firm will provide on request a list of dietetic products which can be ordered, as well as a list of retail distributors in a given area.

Wheat, Milk, and Egg-Free Recipes from Mary Alden. Quaker Oats Company, Merchandise Mart Plaza, Chicago, Ill. 60654.

This list is subject to change. Often new products enter the market and old ones are eliminated by their manufacturers.

Low Gluten:

Low-Gluten Diet with Recipes. Mrs. Margaret M. Shaker, 506 Hogarth, Niles, Ohio 44446. Price: $1.50.

Low Gluten Diet with Tested Recipes. A. B. French, M.D. Price $1.00. Contains wheat-, rye-, oat-, and barley-free recipes. A separate list of some packaged and prepared foods by brand names that may be used in modified gluten diet is also available. Make checks payable to A. B. French Intestinal Research Fund and send to Arthur B. French, M.D., West 4642 Clinical Research Unit, University of Michigan Hospital, Ann Arbor, Mich. 48204.

Luncheon with Laurie. Mrs. Carolyn B. Carpenter, 237 Pinewood Lane, Rock Hill, S.C. 29730. Price: $1.75. A collection of wheat-, rye-, and barley-free recipes.

Milk-free:

Allergy Recipes. The American Dietetic Association, 620 North Michigan Avenue, Chicago, Ill. 60611. Price: $.50.

Allergy Recipes from the Blue Flame Kitchen. Metropolitan Utilities District, 1723 Harney Street, Omaha, Neb. 68102. Price: $.50.

Baking for People with Food Allergies. Superintendent of Documents, U.S. Government Printing Office, Washington, D.C. 20402. Price: $.10.

Cooking with Imagination for Special Diets. Grocery Store Products Company, West Chester, Pa. 19380.

Easy, Appealing Milk-Free Recipes. Mead Johnson & Company, Evansville, Ind. 47221.

Good Recipes to Brighten the Allergy Diet. Best Foods, A Division of CPC International, Inc., Dept. AB, Englewood Cliffs, N.J. 07632. Free.

Jolly Joan, Ener-G Foods, Inc., Seattle, Wash. 98134. Various recipes available.

Loma Linda Foods. Riverside, Calif. 92505. Various recipes available.

125 Great Recipes for Allergy Diets and *Helps for Allergies.* Good Housekeeping Institute, 959 Eighth Avenue, New York, N.Y. 10019. Prices: $.50 and $.10.

Recipes for the Allergic Individual. Kannengiesser & Company, 76 Ninth Avenue, New York, N.Y. 10011. Free.

Recipes for Using Mull-Soy in Milk-Free Diets. Borden's Prescription Products Division. Free.

Recipes for Using Soya Bean Powder. Fearn Soya Foods, Melrose Park, Ill. 60160.

Wheat-free:

Allergy Recipes. The American Dietetic Association, 620 North Michigan Avenue, Chicago, Ill. 60611. Price: $.50.

Allergy Recipes from the Blue Flame Kitchen. Metropolitan Utilities District, 1723 Harney Street, Omaha, Neb. 68102. Price: $.50.

Baking for People with Food Allergies. Superintendent of Documents, U.S. Government Printing Office, Washington, D.C. 20402. Price: $.10.

Cooking with Imagination for Special Diets. Grocery Store Products Company, West Chester, Pa. 19380.

Good Recipes to Brighten the Allergy Diet. Best Foods, A Division of CPC International, Inc., Dept. AB, Englewood Cliffs, N.J. 07632. Free.

Jolly Joan, Ener-G Foods, Inc., Seattle, Wash. 98134. Various recipes available.

Loma Linda Foods. Riverside, Calif. 92505. Various recipes available.

Low-Gluten Diet with Recipes. Mrs. Margaret Shaker, 506 Hogarth, Niles, Ohio 44446. Price: $1.50.

Luncheon with Laurie. Mrs. Carolyn B. Carpenter, 237 Pinewood Lane, Rock Hill, S.C. 29730. Price: $1.75.

125 Great Recipes for Allergy Diets, and *Helps for Allergies.* Good Housekeeping Institute, 959 Eighth Avenue, New York, N.Y. 10019. Prices: $.50 and $.10.

Recipes for the Allergic Individual. Kannengiesser & Company, 76 Ninth Avenue, New York, N.Y. 10011. Free.

Egg-free:

Allergy Recipes. The American Dietetic Association, 620 North Michigan Avenue, Chicago, Ill. 60611. Price: $.50.

Allergy Recipes from the Blue Flame Kitchen. Metropolitan Utilities District, 1723 Harney Street, Omaha, Neb. 68102. Price: $.50

Baking for People with Food Allergies. Superintendent of Documents, U.S. Government Printing Office, Washington, D.C. 20402.

Cooking with Imagination for Special Diets. Grocery Store Products Company, West Chester, Pa. 19380.

Good Recipes to Brighten the Allergy Diet. Best Foods, A Division of CPC International, Inc., Dept. AB, Englewood Cliffs, N.J. 07632. Free.

Helps for Allergies, 125 Great Recipes for Allergy Diets, and *Helps for Allergies (Childhood Allergies).* Good Housekeeping Institute, 959 Eighth Avenue, New York, N.Y. 10019. Prices: $.10, $.50, and $.10.

Jolly Joan, Ener-G Foods, Inc. Seattle, Wash. 98134. Various recipes available.

Loma Linda Foods. Riverside, Calif. 92505. Various recipes available.

Recipes for the Allergic Individual. Kannengiesser & Company, 76 Ninth Avenue, New York, N.Y. 10011. Free.

HEINZ BABY FOODS

The following allergy-free baby foods are manufactured by Heinz.*

CORN-FREE JUNIOR FOODS

Fruits
Apples and Pears
Applesauce
Applesauce and Apricots
Peaches
Pears
Pears and Pineapple

Vegetables
Carrots
Green Beans
Sweet Potatoes

Meats
Beef and Beef Broth
Chicken and Chicken Broth
Chicken Sticks
Lamb and Lamb Broth
Veal and Veal Broth

CORN-FREE INSTANT CEREALS

Barley
High Protein

Oatmeal
Rice

CORN-FREE STRAINED FOODS

Fruits
Apples and Pears
Applesauce
Applesauce and Apricots
Peaches
Pears
Pears and Pineapple

Juices
Apple
Apple-Apricot
Apple-Cherry
Apple-Grape
Apple-Pineapple
Apple-Prune
Mixed Fruit
Orange
Orange-Apple-Banana
Orange-Pineapple

HEINZ BABY FOODS (*continued*)

Meats and Egg Yolks
Beef and Beef Broth
Chicken and Chicken Broth
Egg Yolks
Ham and Ham Broth
Lamb and Lamb Broth
Liver and Liver Broth
Pork and Pork Broth
Turkey and Turkey Broth
Veal and Veal Broth

Breakfasts
Mixed Cereal with Apples and
   Bananas
Oatmeal with Apples and Bananas
Rice Cereal with Apples and
   Bananas

Vegetables
Beets
Carrots
Green Beans
Squash
Sweet Potatoes

WHEAT-FREE JUNIOR FOODS

Fruits
Apples and Cranberries with
   Tapioca
Apples and Pears
Applesauce
Applesauce and Apricots
Apricots with Tapioca
Bananas and Pineapple with
   Tapioca
Cottage Cheese with Bananas
Peaches
Pears
Pears and Pineapple

Meats
Beef and Beef Broth
Chicken and Chicken Broth
Chicken Sticks
Lamb and Lamb Broth
Meat Sticks
Veal and Veal Broth

High Meat Dinners
Beef with Vegetables and Cereal
Chicken with Vegetables
Ham with Vegetables
Turkey with Vegetables
Veal with Vegetables

Dinners and Soups
Chicken Soup
Vegetables and Bacon
Vegetables and Beef

Vegetables
Carrots
Creamed Corn
Creamed Peas
Green Beans
Mixed Vegetables
Sweet Potatoes

Desserts
Custard Pudding
Fruit Dessert
Pineapple Orange Dessert
Tutti Frutti

WHEAT-FREE INSTANT CEREALS

Barley   Rice
Oatmeal

WHEAT-FREE STRAINED FOODS

Fruits

Apples and Cranberries
Apples and Pears
Applesauce
Applesauce and Pears
Apricots with Tapioca
Bananas and Pineapple
Bananas with Tapioca
Cottage Cheese with Bananas
Peaches
Pears
Pears and Pineapple
Plums with Tapioca
Prunes with Tapioca

Juices

Apple
Apple-Apricot
Apple-Cherry
Apple-Grape
Apple-Pineapple
Apple-Prune
Mixed Fruit
Orange
Orange-Apple-Banana
Orange-Pineapple

Meats and Egg Yolks

Beef and Beef Broth
Chicken and Chicken Broth
Egg Yolks
Ham and Ham Broth
Lamb and Lamb Broth
Liver and Liver Broth
Pork and Pork Broth
Turkey and Turkey Broth
Veal and Veal Broth

High Meat Dinners

Beef with Vegetables
Chicken with Vegetables
Ham with Vegetables
Turkey with Vegetables
Veal with Vegetables

Breakfasts, Dinners and Soups

Cereal, Egg Yolks and Bacon
Chicken Soup
Oatmeal with Apples and Bananas
Rice Cereal with Apples and
    Bananas
Vegetables and Bacon
Vegetables and Beef
Vegetables and Ham with Bacon
Vegetables and Lamb

Vegetables

Beets
Carrots
Creamed Corn
Creamed Peas
Green Beans
Mixed Vegetables
Squash
Sweet Potatoes

Desserts

Custard Pudding
Fruit Dessert
Pineapple Orange Dessert
Tutti Frutti

HEINZ BABY FOODS (continued)

MILK-FREE JUNIOR FOODS

Fruits
Apples and Cranberries with
   Tapioca
Apples and Pears
Applesauce
Applesauce and Apricots
Apricots with Tapioca
Bananas and Pineapple with
   Tapioca
Peaches
Pears
Pears and Pineapple

Meats
Beef and Beef Broth
Chicken and Chicken Broth
Lamb and Lamb Broth
Veal and Veal Broth

High Meat Dinners
Beef with Vegetables and Cereal
Chicken with Vegetables
Ham with Vegetables

Breakfasts, Dinners and Soups
Egg Noodles and Beef
Macaroni, Tomatoes, Beef and
   Bacon
Vegetables and Bacon
Vegetables and Beef
Vegetables, Dumplings, Beef and
   Bacon

Vegetables
Carrots
Green Beans
Mixed Vegetables
Sweet Potatoes

Desserts
Apple Pie
Banana Pie
Fruit Dessert
Peach Pie
Pineapple Orange Dessert

MILK-FREE INSTANT CEREALS

Barley
Mixed

Oatmeal
Rice

MILK-FREE STRAINED FOODS

Fruits
Apples and Cranberries
Apples and Pears
Applesauce
Applesauce and Apricots
Apricots with Tapioca
Bananas and Pineapple

Bananas with Tapioca
Peaches
Pears
Pears and Pineapple
Plums with Tapioca
Prunes with Tapioca

Juices
Apple
Apple-Apricot
Apple-Cherry
Apple-Grape
Apple-Pineapple
Apple-Prune
Mixed Fruit
Orange
Orange-Apple-Banana
Orange-Pineapple

Meats and Egg Yolks
Beef and Beef Broth
Chicken and Chicken Broth
Egg Yolks
Ham and Ham Broth
Lamb and Lamb Broth
Liver and Liver Broth
Pork and Pork Broth
Turkey and Turkey Broth
Veal and Veal Broth

High Meat Dinners
Beef with Vegetables
Chicken with Vegetables
Ham with Vegetables
Veal with Vegetables

Breakfasts, Dinners and Soups
Beef and Egg Noodles
Mixed Cereal with Apples and
  Bananas
Oatmeal with Apples and Bananas
Rice Cereal with Apples and
  Bananas
Vegetables and Bacon
Vegetables and Beef
Vegetables and Ham with Bacon
Vegetables, Dumplings, Beef and
  Bacon

Vegetables
Beets
Carrots
Green Beans
Mixed Vegetables
Squash
Sweet Potatoes

Desserts
Apple Pie
Banana Pie
Fruit Dessert
Peach Pie
Pineapple Orange Dessert

CITRUS FRUIT-FREE JUNIOR FOODS

Fruits
Apples and Cranberries with
  Tapioca
Apples and Pears
Applesauce
Applesauce and Apricots
Apricots with Tapioca
Peaches
Pears and Pineapple

Meats
Beef and Beef Broth
Chicken and Chicken Broth
Chicken Sticks
Lamb and Lamb Broth
Meat Sticks
Veal and Veal Broth

High Meat Dinners
Beef with Vegetables and Cereal
Chicken with Vegetables
Ham with Vegetables
Turkey with Vegetables
Veal with Vegetables

HEINZ BABY FOODS (*continued*)

Breakfasts, Dinners and Soups
Cereal, Eggs and Bacon
Chicken Noodle Dinner
Egg Noodles and Beef
Macaroni, Tomatoes, Beef and
  Bacon
Vegetables and Bacon
Vegetables and Beef
Vegetables and Ham with Bacon
Vegetables and Lamb
Vegetables, Dumplings, Beef and
  Bacon
Vegetables, Egg Noodles and
  Chicken
Vegetables, Egg Noodles and
  Turkey

Vegetables
Carrots
Creamed Corn
Creamed Peas
Green Beans
Mixed Vegetables
Sweet Potatoes

Desserts
Apple Pie
Custard Pudding
Peach Pie

CITRUS FRUIT-FREE INSTANT CEREALS

Barley
High Protein
Mixed

Oatmeal
Rice

CITRUS FRUIT-FREE STRAINED FOODS

Fruits
Apples and Cranberries
Apples and Pears
Applesauce
Applesauce and Apricots
Apricots with Tapioca
Peaches
Pears
Pears and Pineapple
Plums with Tapioca
Prunes with Tapioca

Juices
Apple
Apple-Apricot
Apple-Cherry
Apple-Grape
Apple-Pineapple
Apple-Prune

Meats and Egg Yolks

Beef and Beef Broth
Chicken and Chicken Broth
Egg Yolks
Ham and Ham Broth
Lamb and Lamb Broth
Liver and Liver Broth
Pork and Pork Broth
Turkey and Turkey Broth
Veal and Veal Broth

High Meat Dinners

Beef with Vegetables
Chicken with Vegetables
Ham with Vegetables
Turkey with Vegetables
Veal with Vegetables

Vegetables

Beets
Carrots
Creamed Corn
Creamed Peas
Green Beans
Mixed Vegetables
Squash
Sweet Potatoes

Breakfasts, Dinners and Soups

Beef and Egg Noodles
Cereal, Egg Yolks and Bacon
Chicken Noodle Dinner
Chicken Soup
Macaroni, Tomatoes, Beef and
  Bacon
Mixed Cereal with Apples and
  Bananas
Oatmeal with Apples and Bananas
Rice Cereal with Apples and
  Bananas
Vegetables and Bacon
Vegetables and Beef
Vegetables and Ham with Bacon
Vegetables and Lamb
Vegetables, Dumplings, Beef and
  Bacon
Vegetables, Egg Noodles and
  Chicken
Vegetables, Egg Noodles and
  Turkey

Desserts

Apple Pie
Custard Pudding
Peach Pie

GLUTEN-FREE JUNIOR FOODS

Fruits

Apples and Cranberries with
  Tapioca
Apples and Pears
Applesauce
Applesauce and Apricots
Apricots with Tapioca
Bananas and Pineapple with
  Tapioca
Cottage Cheese with Bananas
Peaches
Pears
Pears and Pineapple

Meats

Beef and Beef Broth
Chicken and Chicken Broth
Chicken Sticks
Lamb and Lamb Broth
Meat Sticks
Veal and Veal Broth

High Meat Dinners

Ham with Vegetables
Turkey with Vegetables

HEINZ BABY FOODS (*continued*)

Vegetables
Carrots
Creamed Corn
Creamed Peas
Green Beans
Mixed Vegetables
Sweet Potatoes

Desserts
Custard Pudding
Fruit Dessert
Pineapple Orange Dessert
Tutti Frutti

GLUTEN-FREE INSTANT CEREALS

Rice

GLUTEN-FREE STRAINED FOODS

Fruits
Apples and Cranberries
Apples and Pears
Applesauce
Applesauce and Apricots
Apricots with Tapioca
Bananas and Pineapple
Bananas with Tapioca
Cottage Cheese with Bananas
Peaches
Pears
Pears and Pineapple
Plums with Tapioca
Prunes with Tapioca

Juices
Apple
Apple-Apricot
Apple-Cherry
Apple-Grape
Apple-Pineapple
Apple-Prune
Mixed Fruit
Orange
Orange-Apple-Banana
Orange-Pineapple

Meats and Egg Yolks
Beef and Beef Broth
Chicken and Chicken Broth
Egg Yolks
Ham and Ham Broth
Lamb and Lamb Broth
Liver and Liver Broth
Pork and Pork Broth
Turkey and Turkey Broth
Veal and Veal Broth

High Meat Dinners
Beef with Vegetables
Chicken with Vegetables
Ham and Vegetables
Turkey with Vegetables
Veal with Vegetables

Breakfasts, Dinners and Soups
Chicken Soup
Vegetables and Bacon
Vegetables and Ham with Bacon
Vegetables and Lamb

Vegetables
Beets
Carrots
Creamed Corn
Creamed Peas
Green Beans
Squash
Sweet Potatoes

Desserts
Custard Pudding
Fruit Dessert
Pineapple Orange Dessert
Tutti Frutti

EGG-FREE JUNIOR FOODS

Fruits
Apples and Cranberries with
  Tapioca
Apples and Pears
Applesauce
Applesauce and Apricots
Apricots with Tapioca
Bananas and Pineapple with
  Tapioca
Cottage Cheese with Bananas
Peaches
Pears
Pears and Pineapple

Meats
Beef and Beef Broth
Chicken and Chicken Broth
Chicken Sticks
Lamb and Lamb Broth
Meat Sticks
Veal and Veal Broth

High Meat Dinners
Beef with Vegetables and Cereal
Chicken with Vegetables
Ham with Vegetables
Turkey with Vegetables
Veal with Vegetables

Breakfasts, Dinners and Soups
Macaroni, Tomatoes, Beef and
  Bacon
Vegetables and Bacon
Vegetables and Beef
Vegetables and Ham with Bacon
Vegetables and Lamb

Vegetables
Carrots
Creamed Corn
Creamed Peas
Green Beans
Mixed Vegetables
Sweet Potatoes

Desserts
Apple Pie
Banana Pie
Fruit Dessert
Peach Pie

Instant Cereals
Barley
High Protein
Mixed
Oatmeal
Rice

HEINZ BABY FOODS (*continued*)

EGG-FREE STRAINED FOODS

Fruits
Apples and Cranberries
Apples and Pears
Applesauce
Applesauce and Apricots
Apricots with Tapioca
Bananas with Tapioca
Bananas and Pineapple
Cottage Cheese with Bananas
Peaches
Pears
Pears and Pineapple
Plums with Tapioca
Prunes with Tapioca

Juices
Apple
Apple-Apricot
Apple-Cherry
Apple-Grape
Apple-Pineapple
Apple-Prune
Mixed Fruit
Orange
Orange-Apple-Banana
Orange-Pineapple

Meats
Beef and Beef Broth
Chicken and Chicken Broth
Ham and Ham Broth
Lamb and Lamb Broth
Liver and Liver Broth
Pork and Pork Broth
Turkey and Turkey Broth
Veal and Veal Broth

High Meat Dinners
Beef with Vegetables
Chicken with Vegetables
Ham with Vegetables
Turkey with Vegetables
Veal with Vegetables

Breakfasts, Dinners and Soups
Chicken Soup
Macaroni, Tomatoes, Beef and
  Bacon
Mixed Cereal with Apples and
  Bananas
Oatmeal with Apples and Bananas
Rice Cereal with Apples and
  Bananas
Vegetables and Bacon
Vegetables and Beef
Vegetables and Ham with Bacon
Vegetables and Lamb

Vegetables
Beets
Carrots
Creamed Corn
Creamed Peas
Green Beans
Mixed Vegetables
Squash
Sweet Potatoes

Desserts
Apple Pie
Banana Pie
Fruit Dessert
Peach Pie

MILK, WHEAT, EGG AND CITRUS FRUIT-FREE JUNIOR FOODS

Fruits
Apples and Cranberries with
  Tapioca
Apples and Pears
Applesauce
Applesauce and Apricots
Apricots with Tapioca
Peaches
Pears
Pears and Pineapple

Meats
Beef and Beef Broth
Chicken and Chicken Broth
Lamb and Lamb Broth
Veal and Veal Broth

High Meat Dinners
Beef with Vegetables and Cereal
Chicken with Vegetables
Ham with Vegetables
Veal with Vegetables

Dinners
Vegetables and Bacon
Vegetables and Beef

Vegetables
Carrots
Green Beans
Mixed Vegetables
Sweet Potatoes

MILK, WHEAT, EGG, AND CITRUS FRUIT-FREE INSTANT CEREALS

Barley
Oatmeal

Rice

MILK, WHEAT, EGG AND CITRUS FRUIT-FREE STRAINED FOODS

Fruits
Apples and Cranberries
Apples and Pears
Applesauce
Applesauce and Apricots
Apricots with Tapioca
Peaches
Pears
Pears and Pineapple
Plums with Tapioca
Prunes with Tapioca

Juices
Apple
Apple-Apricot
Apple-Cherry
Apple-Grape
Apple-Pineapple
Apple-Prune

Meats
Beef and Beef Broth
Chicken and Chicken Broth
Ham and Ham Broth
Lamb and Lamb Broth
Liver and Liver Broth
Pork and Pork Broth
Turkey and Turkey Broth
Veal and Veal Broth

High Meat Dinners
Beef with Vegetables
Chicken with Vegetables
Ham with Vegetables
Veal with Vegetables

HEINZ BABY FOODS (*continued*)

Breakfasts, Dinners and Soups
Oatmeal with Apples and Bananas
Rice Cereal with Apples and
   Bananas
Vegetables and Bacon
Vegetables and Beef
Vegetables and Ham with Bacon

Vegetables
Beets
Carrots
Green Beans
Mixed Vegetables
Squash
Sweet Potatoes

BEECH-NUT BABY FOODS

The following allergy-free baby foods are manufactured by Beech-Nut.

WHEAT-FREE STRAINED FOODS

Packaged Cereals
Rice Cereal
Oatmeal Cereal
Honey Flavored Rice
Honey Flavored Oatmeal

Juices
Apple
Apple-Cherry
Apple-Grape
Orange
Orange-Apple
Orange-Apricot
Orange-Banana
Orange-Pineapple
Prune-Orange
Mixed Fruit

Meats and Egg Yolks
Beef
Chicken
Ham
Lamb
Pork
Turkey
Veal
Egg Yolks
Egg Yolks and Bacon

High Meat Dinners
Beef
Chicken
Ham
Turkey
Veal

Vegetables
Carrots
Carrots in Butter Sauce
Creamed Corn
Garden Vegetables
Green Beans
Peas
Peas in Butter Sauce
Squash
Squash in Butter Sauce
Sweet Potatoes
Sweet Potatoes in Butter Sauce

Dinners and Soups
Turkey Rice Dinner
Vegetable Soup
Vegetables and Bacon
Vegetables and Beef
Vegetables and Lamb
Vegetables and Liver
Oatmeal with Fruit

Desserts

Caramel Pudding
Peach Melba
Apple Betty
Chocolate Custard Pudding
Custard Pudding

Fruit Dessert with Tapioca
Orange Pineapple Dessert
Pineapple Dessert
Creamed Cottage Cheese with
   Pineapple Juice

EGG-FREE STRAINED FOODS

Packaged Cereals

Rice Cereal
Oatmeal Cereal
Mixed Cereal
Hi-Protein Cereal
Honey Flavored Rice
Honey Flavored Oatmeal
Honey Flavored Mixed

Juices

Apple
Apple-Cherry
Apple-Grape
Orange
Orange-Apple
Orange-Apricot
Orange-Banana
Orange-Pineapple
Prune-Orange
Mixed Fruit

Meats and Egg Yolks

Beef
Chicken
Ham
Lamb
Pork
Turkey
Veal

High Meat Dinners

Beef
Chicken
Ham
Turkey
Veal

Vegetables

Carrots
Carrots in Butter Sauce
Creamed Corn
Garden Vegetables
Green Beans
Green Beans in Butter Sauce
Peas
Peas in Butter Sauce
Squash
Squash in Butter Sauce
Sweet Potatoes
Sweet Potatoes in Butter Sauce

Dinners and Soups

Chicken with Vegetables
Vegetable Soup
Turkey Rice Dinner
Vegetables and Bacon
Vegetables and Beef
Vegetables and Ham
Vegetables and Lamb
Vegetables and Liver
Oatmeal with Fruit
Mixed Cereal with Fruit

Desserts

Apple Betty
Fruit Dessert with Tapioca
Creamed Cottage Cheese with
   Pineapple Juice
Peach Melba

BEECH-NUT BABY FOODS (*continued*)

MILK-FREE STRAINED FOODS

Packaged Cereals
Oatmeal
Rice Cereal
Mixed Cereal
Hi-Protein Cereal
Honey Flavored Oatmeal
Honey Flavored Mixed
Honey Flavored Rice

Juices
Apple
Apple-Cherry
Apple-Grape
Orange
Orange-Apple
Orange-Apricot
Orange-Banana
Orange-Pineapple
Prune-Orange
Mixed Fruit

Meats and Egg Yolks
Beef
Chicken
Ham
Lamb
Pork
Turkey
Veal
Egg Yolks
Egg Yolks and Bacon

High Meat Dinners
Beef
Chicken
Ham
Turkey
Veal

Vegetables
Carrots
Garden Vegetables
Green Beans
Peas
Squash
Sweet Potatoes

Dinners and Soups
Chicken with Vegetables
Vegetable Soup
Beef and Noodles
Chicken Noodle Dinner
Turkey Rice Dinner
Vegetables and Bacon
Vegetables and Beef
Vegetables and Lamb
Vegetables and Liver
Oatmeal with Fruit
Mixed Cereal with Fruit

Desserts
Fruit Dessert with Tapioca
Orange Pineapple Dessert
Peach Melba

CITRUS FRUIT-FREE STRAINED FOODS

Packaged Cereals
Rice Cereal
Oatmeal Cereal
Mixed Cereal
Hi-Protein Cereal
Honey Flavored Rice
Honey Flavored Mixed
Honey Flavored Oatmeal

Juices
Apple
Apple-Cherry
Apple-Grape

Meats and Egg Yolks
Beef
Chicken
Ham
Lamb
Pork
Turkey
Veal
Egg Yolks
Egg Yolks and Bacon

High Meat Dinners
Beef
Chicken
Ham
Turkey
Veal

Vegetables
Carrots
Carrots in Butter Sauce
Creamed Corn
Garden Vegetables
Green Beans
Green Beans in Butter Sauce
Peas
Peas in Butter Sauce
Squash
Squash in Butter Sauce
Sweet Potatoes
Sweet Potatoes in Butter Sauce

Dinners and Soups
Chicken with Vegetables
Vegetable Soup
Beef and Noodle Dinner
Macaroni, Tomato Sauce, Beef and
    Bacon Dinner
Turkey Rice Dinner
Vegetables and Bacon
Vegetables and Beef
Vegetables and Ham
Vegetables and Lamb
Vegetables and Liver
Cereal, Egg Yolks and Bacon

Desserts
Custard Pudding
Chocolate Custard Dessert
Pineapple Dessert
Creamed Cottage Cheese with
    Pineapple Juice
Apple Betty
Caramel Pudding
Peach Melba

WHEAT-EGG-MILK-CITRUS FRUIT-FREE FOODS

Packaged Cereals
Rice Cereal
Honey Flavored Rice
Honey Flavored Mixed
Honey Flavored Oatmeal

Juices
Apple
Apple-Cherry
Apple-Grape

Meats and Egg Yolks
Beef
Chicken
Ham
Lamb
Pork
Turkey
Veal

BEECH-NUT BABY FOODS (*continued*)

High Meat Dinners
Beef
Chicken
Ham
Turkey
Veal

Vegetables
Carrots
Garden Vegetables
Green Beans
Peas
Squash
Sweet Potatoes

Dinners and Soups
Turkey Rice, Vegetable and Bacon
Vegetable Soup
Vegetables and Beef
Vegetables and Lamb
Vegetables and Liver

Fruits
Applesauce
Applesauce and Cherries
Applesauce and Raspberries
Apples and Apricots
Apricots with Tapioca
Bananas with Tapioca
Bananas and Pineapple with
   Tapioca
Peaches
Pears
Pears and Pineapple
Plums with Tapioca
Prunes with Tapioca

WHEAT-FREE JUNIOR FOODS

Meats and Egg Yolks
Beef
Chicken
Chicken Sticks
Meat Sticks
Lamb
Pork
Turkey
Veal

High Meat Dinners
Beef
Chicken
Ham
Turkey
Veal

Vegetables
Carrots
Carrots in Butter Sauce
Peas in Butter Sauce
Green Beans
Squash
Squash in Butter Sauce
Sweet Potatoes
Sweet Potatoes in Butter Sauce
Green Beans in Butter Sauce

Dinners and Soups
Vegetable Soup
Split Peas, Vegetable and Ham
Turkey Rice Dinner
Vegetables and Bacon
Vegetables and Beef
Vegetables and Lamb
Vegetables and Liver

Desserts
Peach Melba
Caramel Pudding
Apple Betty
Custard Pudding

Fruit Dessert with Tapioca
Tropical Fruit Dessert
Banana Dessert
Creamed Cottage Cheese with
    Pineapple

EGG-FREE JUNIOR FOODS

Meats and Egg Yolks
Beef
Chicken
Chicken Sticks
Meat Sticks
Lamb
Pork
Turkey
Veal

High Meat Dinners
Beef
Chicken
Ham
Turkey
Veal

Vegetables
Carrots
Carrots in Butter Sauce
Peas in Butter Sauce
Green Beans
Green Beans in Butter Sauce
Squash
Squash in Butter Sauce
Sweet Potatoes
Sweet Potatoes in Butter Sauce

Dinners and Soups
Chicken with Vegetables
Vegetable Soup
Macaroni and Bacon with
    Vegetables
Macaroni and Beef with Vegetables
Spaghetti, Tomato Sauce and Beef
Split Peas, Vegetables and Ham
Turkey Rice Dinner
Vegetables and Bacon
Vegetables and Beef
Vegetables and Lamb
Vegetables and Liver

Desserts
Apple Betty
Banana Dessert
Fruit Dessert with Tapioca
Tropical Fruit Dessert
Creamed Cottage Cheese with
    Pineapple
Peach Melba

Fruits
Applesauce
Applesauce and Cherries
Applesauce and Raspberries
Apples and Apricots
Peaches
Apples with Tapioca
Pears
Pears and Pineapple
Plums with Tapioca
Prunes with Tapioca
Banana and Pineapple with Tapioca

BEECH-NUT BABY FOODS (*continued*)

MILK-FREE JUNIOR FOODS

Meats and Egg Yolks
Beef
Chicken
Lamb
Pork
Turkey
Veal

High Meat Dinners
Beef
Chicken
Ham
Turkey
Veal

Vegetables
Carrots
Green Beans
Squash
Sweet Potatoes

Dinners and Soups
Chicken with Vegetables
Vegetable Soup
Beef and Noodles
Chicken Noodle Dinner
Macaroni and Beef with Vegetables
Turkey Rice Dinner
Vegetables and Beef
Vegetables and Lamb
Vegetables and Liver

Desserts
Banana Dessert
Fruit Dessert with Tapioca
Tropical Fruit Dessert
Peach Melba

CITRUS FRUIT-FREE JUNIOR FOODS

Meats and Egg Yolks
Beef
Chicken
Chicken Sticks
Meat Sticks
Lamb
Turkey
Pork
Veal

High Meat Dinners
Beef
Chicken
Ham
Turkey
Veal

Vegetables
Carrots
Carrots in Butter Sauce
Green Beans
Squash
Squash in Butter Sauce
Sweet Potatoes in Butter Sauce
Sweet Potatoes
Green Beans in Butter Sauce
Peas in Butter Sauce

Dinners and Soups
Chicken with Vegetables
Cereal, Egg Yolks and Bacon
Vegetable Soup
Beef and Noodles
Chicken and Noodles
Lamb and Noodles
Macaroni and Bacon with
    Vegetables
Macaroni and Beef with Vegetables
Spaghetti, Tomato Sauce and Beef
Split Peas, Vegetables and Ham
Turkey Rice Dinner
Vegetables and Bacon
Vegetables and Beef
Vegetables and Lamb
Vegetables and Liver

Desserts
Custard Pudding
Creamed Cottage Cheese with
    Pineapple Juice
Apple Betty
Caramel Pudding
Peach Melba

Fruits
Applesauce
Applesauce and Cherries
Applesauce and Raspberries
Apples and Apricots
Apricots with Tapioca
Peaches
Pears
Pears and Pineapple
Plums with Tapioca
Prunes with Tapioca

WHEAT-EGG-MILK-CITRUS FRUIT-FREE JUNIOR FOODS

Meats and Egg Yolks
Beef
Chicken
Lamb
Pork
Turkey
Veal

High Meat Dinners
Beef
Chicken
Ham
Turkey
Veal

Vegetables
Carrots
Green Beans
Squash
Sweet Potatoes

Dinners and Soups
Vegetable Soup
Turkey Rice Dinner
Vegetables and Beef
Vegetables and Lamb
Vegetables and Liver

12 Epilogue

Now that we have come to the end of this book, what should the parents of an atopic child have learned from it? Certain principles are basic and they cannot do without them.

1. An atopic baby must be kept clean to prevent eczema and infection. He must avoid moisture, bacteria, detergents, bleaches, or smells, especially under his diapers. To do that, he must have his skin made soft with baby oil, and dry with baby powder. He must be sponged a few times daily during the first weeks, and later tub-bathed once daily. Strong soaps with disinfectants must never be used on him but mild and nonallergenic soaps. This sort of cleanliness makes him feel well, and well taken care of.

2. An atopic child must get accustomed to healthy and hypoallergenic foods, beginning when he is a baby. Breastfeeding is very important to him. It gives him a healthy outlook on life and less trouble with milk allergies. Among solid foods some cereals like corn are very allergenic, and they should be avoided altogether, while rice is hypoallergenic and should be indulged in. Of all the meats, the child should be encouraged to eat lamb, and among the oils he should choose olive. He must avoid complicated recipes, shellfish, chocolate, nuts, fresh fruit in general and exotic fruits in particular. His parents must not forget his vitamins, and should not worry about missing essential food items from his diet; the substitutes suggested in this book contain all the ingredients he needs to develop normally. He needs his foods to thrive on, not to get sick on. His parents must encourage him to develop the good eating habits that they expect from their other children.

3. What should the atopic child wear? He must avoid synthetics, wools, rayon, Orlon, and so on and should use soft cottons on his skin.

4. An atopic child should never have a pet. He should avoid the attachment that he may form to a dog, a cat, or a canary; he does not need the trauma of separation from his pet later on. He may be encouraged to have nonallergenic rubber or wooden animal substitutes.

5. How should parents familiarize themselves with a child's allergies? They must get a book like this one and get acquainted with eczema, hay fever, allergic rhinitis, and asthma, and ignore the rare allergic disorders that will probably never occur in their child. They must leave the complex ailments of the baby to his doctor.

6. When an atopic child falls ill with one of the allergic diseases the parents must keep calm and inspire confidence. Their child is doubly sensitive to his illness, and they have already accepted him as he is now, even before he was conceived. Most likely at least one of the parents has had allergies, and they know what that means. Parents must trust their instinct, and remember that nature is always on their side. In asthma, high temperature eases the disease, while vomiting makes the child get rid of his mucus. Above all, they must not overmedicate, and surely not with complicated drugs. They must avoid penicillin and aspirin at all costs; they must also avoid nose drops with vasoconstrictors and use normal saline in their place. They must not stop a cough with cough suppressants, because mucus brings in bacteria. They must judge vomiting and diarrhea, not from the point of view of indigestion, but rather from that of a food allergy. Rashes have to be exactly diagnosed; there are those that normally pertain to a child, and those that are brought about by allergies.

7. What about the child's environment?

This has to be controlled emotionally and physically.

As far as emotional control is concerned, an atopic child will have the normal fears that any child has, plus the particular ones born out of his allergies. Fear of growing up with a deformed skin in eczema, or fear of strangulation in asthma, are to an atopic child real and actual fears. Parents must learn to handle these fears realistically, yet not with indifference, oversolicitousness or over-permissiveness. They can use toys to help them achieve this aim. Toys are important to the imagination of a child, and much mental and emotional development can be achieved through their use. The atopic child, however, can play only with certain specific toys. Such toys must have smooth contours and no niches that collect dust, be painted with lead-free paints, have no scent, cutting edge, stuffing of cotton or animal hair, buttons, glass, long cords, small screws, or tiny complicated parts. They must be durable, accessible, designed to suit the mentality of the child, and be reasonably priced. They will stimulate his imagination, allay his fears, and distract him from his food and environmental limitations. They have to be changed constantly to fit his age, and at two, as the baby gets to be a little child, the toys have to make him distinguish between what is real and what is imaginary. At around three the child begins to shift from toys to television; there he should watch educational programs like *Sesame Street,* and avoid thrillers and crime shows. The change of toys or TV programs must continue to ensure a healthy and normal physical and emotional growth. The child must be made to realize that he is operating within his limits and that he has the capacity to change and grow.

Physical control means control of inhalants present in the bedroom, the temperature of that room, its humidity, its barometric pressure, and its air pollution. The inhalants are to be eliminated because the child spends half of his life in that room. Particles of house dust, feathers, molds, pollen, odors, and so forth have to be removed mechanically through filtration or electronically through precipitation.

The humidity of the room is to be measured in terms of the percentage of water vapor actually present in the room as compared to the amount the room can actually hold. This is the relative humidity of the bedroom, and its optimum level is about 40 percent. This level can be maintained through the use of humidifiers that have a humidistat. Adequate humidification is a necessity and not a luxury.

Air pollution is the presence in the air of particles of dust, chemicals, fumes, mists, fog, smoke, smog, vapors, gases, airborne pollen, and living organisms. Industrial complexes and the use of the car are the main source of this trouble. An asthmatic child cannot inhale this dirty air and has to be relocated in a dry, non-polluted area.

8. What about consulting a pediatric allergist?

A child with multiple allergies needs the services of a pediatric allergist. Before seeking one out, the parents must consult with the family physician, who will make a house call to see for himself whether a dog, a cat, or a canary are present in the house, to examine the bedroom of the baby for dust and dampness, and to assess the emotional balance of the different members of the family. He will then refer his findings, by filling out a form like the following, to the pediatric allergist, who will begin with a clear picture of the history of the child, his environment, and his emotions.

If the child has bronchial asthma, the physician must add to the form these facts: the influence of dampness, dryness, clouds, sun, rain, snow, or smog on the attacks; the symptoms that accompany the attack, such as shortness of breath, wheeze, cough, temperature, and whether these are mild, moderate or severe; the daily activity of the child during attacks and whether this is normal, restricted, or bedridden; the medication that is usually given to stop the attacks; and the diet of the child during the attacks.

When the pediatric allergist's work-up is done, the parents must ask for the diagnosis of the child's illness and a list of the child's main allergens, whether they be pollen, animals, molds, insects, foods, and so forth. They must keep that list with the records of the child and send a copy of it to the school nurse.

Referring physician	Address	Phone

Child's name	Address	Phone

Chief complaint

Present illness

The child's family history in allergy: asthma, eczema, hives, nasal allergy, migraine, or digestive trouble in father, mother, brothers, sisters, uncles and aunts.

The child's allergic history:
Birth date   Birth wt.   Feeding (milk)

Vomiting   Diarrhea   Eczema   Rhinitis   Asthma

Known allergies of the child to foods

Known allergies of the child to drugs

Known allergies of the child to animals

Drugs previously used by the child and their effect.

Previous allergy tests, X-rays, and laboratory findings.

Home environment, and child's bedroom: carpeting, pets, dampness, heating system, hobbies.

Glossary

Allergen. A substance toward which one has antipathy. Allergens may cause an illness when they are eaten (foods), inhaled (dust), or when they come in contact with the skin (cosmetics).

Allergy. A feeling of antipathy or repugnance to a substance found normally in the environment. Clinically, this antipathy shows up as a disease in which one sneezes, has difficulty in breathing, itches, has diarrhea, and so forth.

Alveoli. The tiny air sacs in the lungs where oxygen and carbon dioxide are exchanged.

Amino acid. An organic acid that functions as a block in the structure of a protein.

Ammonia. A pungent and smelly gas synthesized by bacteria from the urine of diapers. In cold weather it becomes an irritative liquid and causes diaper rash.

Anaphylaxis. The most severe and dangerous form of all the allergic reactions.

Angioedema. Giant hives, or an allergic reaction that causes a wheal formation on the skin.

Antibiotic. A substance made by some bacteria that, even in small quantities, can kill other bacteria.

Antibody. A substance called *globulin* that can combine with an allergen to neutralize its toxins, precipitate its bacteria, and in general defend the body against the harmful effects of an antigen.

Antigen. A substance that causes a hypersensitivity allergic reaction and induces the formation of antibodies.

Antitoxin. An antibody that neutralizes the effect of a toxin or a poison. For example, horses are inoculated with the microbe of diphtheria to make them fall sick with it. The blood serum of these horses develops protective diphtheria antitoxins that can be injected into human beings who are sick with diphtheria in order to immunize them against the toxic effects of the disease.

Asthma. A disease marked by episodes of difficult breathing and wheezing.

Atopy. An inherited predisposition to fall sick with one of the allergic diseases.

Bronchial tree. That part of the respiratory tract below the windpipe extending into the lungs, consisting of many subdividing air passages.

Bronchioles. The smallest air passages in the bronchial tree.

Bronchitis. Inflammation of the bronchial tube.

Blocking antibodies. Antibodies that "block" the union of a new antigen to a specific antibody formed previously through a natural exposure to that antigen.

Blocking antibodies are made use of in desensitization. An antigen is injected in increasing doses. The injections form antibodies in the serum, antibodies that have more affinity to the antigen than the antibodies that were formed naturally. If the child is exposed to the same antigen again, no allergic reaction takes place. The new antigens are blocked by the antibodies formed through the desensitizing injections from uniting with the antibodies formed previously through natural exposure to the antigen.

Capillaries. Minute blood vessels forming a network throughout the body.

Cortisone. A hormone isolated from the suprarenal gland, and also prepared synthetically.

Desensitization (or *hyposensitization* or *immunotherapy*). A series of injections designed to diminish sensitivity to an antigen.

Diaphragm. The muscular partition separating the chest from the abdomen.

Eczema. A chronic inflammation in the skin of an allergic child.

Emphysema. A chronic disease of the lungs marked by permanent changes in the alveoli (air passages).

Hay fever. A seasonal allergy of the nose caused by pollen or molds.

Histamine. A chemical released through the interaction of an antigen and its specific antibody.

Hypersensitivity. An abnormal susceptibility to the action of an antigen.

Hyposensitization. See *Desensitization.*

Immunity. The state of being resistant to an allergy or other diseases.

Immunotherapy. See *Desensitization.*

Mold. A growth of minute fungi forming on vegetable or animal matter, commonly seen as a downy or fury coating, and associated with decay.

Mucous membrane. A thin layer of tissue that secretes mucus and lines the nose, lungs, and other organs.

Mucus. A sticky, watery secretion produced by various membranes.

Pollen. The fertilizing element of flowering plants, consisting of fine powdery, yellowish grains, occurring at times in masses like dust.

Respiratory tract. The entire breathing system, from the mouth and nose through the trachea and bronchial trees to the alveoli in the lungs.

Rhinitis. An inflammation of the mucous membrane of the nose.

Serum. The fluid portion of the blood that remains after the blood clots.

Serum sickness. An allergic disease caused by the injection of an immunized horse serum.

Steroids. The hormones of the suprarenal gland and the sex hormones.

Trachea. The windpipe.

Urticaria. The scientific name for hives or itchy blotches on the skin.

Wheezing. Difficult, noisy breathing typical of asthma.

Index